beginner's guide to
body
toning

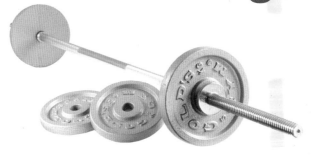

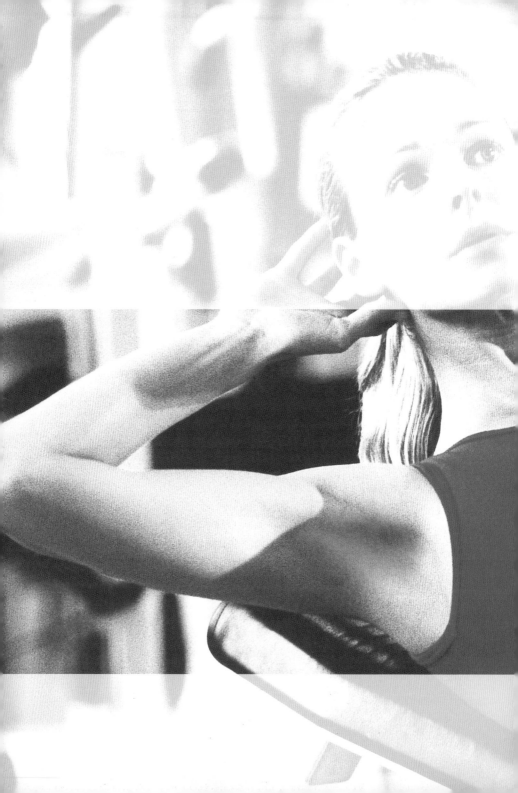

beginner's guide to
body
toning

NATASHA WOLEK

BARRON'S

First edition for the United States,
its territories and dependencies, and
Canada published 2004
by Barron's Educational Series, Inc.

Conceived and created by
Axis Publishing Limited
8c Accommodation Road
London NW11 8ED
www.axispublishing.co.uk

Creative Director: Siân Keogh
Editorial Director: Denis Kennedy
Designer: Axis Design Editions
Managing Editor: Conor Kilgallon
Production Manager: Tim Clarke
Photographer: Mike Good

© 2004 Axis Publishing Limited

All inquiries should be addressed to:
Barron's Educational Series, Inc.
250 Wireless Boulevard
Hauppauge, New York 11788
www.barronseduc.com

Library of Congress Catalog Card No:
2003109362

ISBN 0-7641-2762-4

Printed and bound in China

9 8 7 6 5 4 3 2 1

contents

beginner's guide to **body** toning

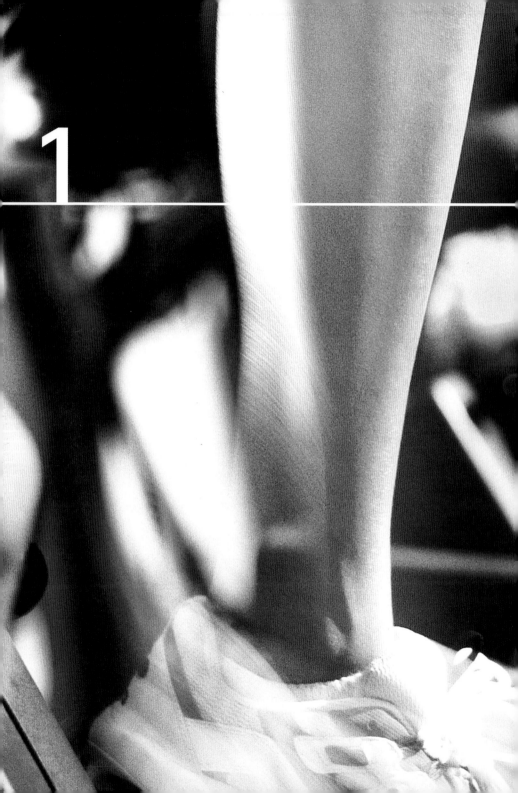

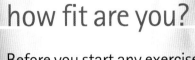

how fit are you?

Before you start any exercise program, you need to become familiar with the information being presented. This chapter will show you how to use this book and identify the people at whom the training levels are aimed. It will also show you the benefits of body toning and guide you through a self-assessment exercise, which will help you to determine your current fitness level.

why tone and sculpt?

Congratulations. By buying this book and reading it, you have made a positive step toward a more active and healthy life. This book is a comprehensive, easy-to-follow guide to toning and sculpting. It uses simple language and clear illustrations, and is packed with information and ideas on how to get fitter and more active.

More and more people are becoming aware of the benefits of exercise and a healthy lifestyle. When used alongside a healthy eating plan and cardiovascular training, toning and sculpting is the most effective way to begin improving your physical appearance—and you don't need to have previous experience to start!

benefits of body toning

Regular exercise has many benefits. Most significantly, it will make your heart and lungs stronger, which will make you feel generally fitter and happier. Exercise reduces the risk of dying prematurely of heart disease; reduces the risk of developing high blood pressure, diabetes, or colon cancer; and helps with weight control. Regular exercise can also provide the following benefits:

▶▶ **increased confidence**   By training hard you will gradually see improvements in how you look and feel. Be proud of your achievements—be it fat loss, increased muscle tone, or improved fitness—and enjoy feeling in control of how you look. By meeting your goals at the gym, you will build confidence that will benefit all areas of your life.

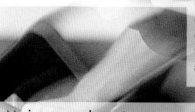

▶▶ **less negative stress**   Negative stress is reduced when exercising and positive stress (known as eustress) is increased. By concentrating on training and enjoying time for yourself, even three times a week, you will release endorphins that will give you increased energy and that feel-good factor. By releasing any negative stress through exercise, you will also feel calmer and more relaxed in day-to-day life.

▶▶ **improved posture**   By learning how to exercise properly, you learn how to sit, how to lift things, and how to stand in everyday life. This can help eliminate lower back pain, which is one of the major causes of absence from work in the western world.

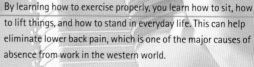

The exercises are straightforward and you can do them anywhere, with or without equipment.

What's more, you don't have to pay lots of money to go to a gym, because many of the exercises you can do at home, and you don't have to stop training when you are traveling. Once you are confident with the basic toning exercises that use your own body weight or light weights, you can start using heavier weights to define and sculpt your body. When you feel ready, you can progress to other types of exercise; alternatively, you may want to take group classes or join a gym to continue your training.

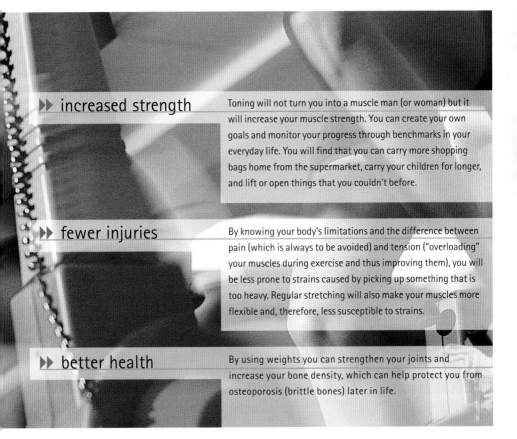

▶▶ increased strength

Toning will not turn you into a muscle man (or woman) but it will increase your muscle strength. You can create your own goals and monitor your progress through benchmarks in your everyday life. You will find that you can carry more shopping bags home from the supermarket, carry your children for longer, and lift or open things that you couldn't before.

▶▶ fewer injuries

By knowing your body's limitations and the difference between pain (which is always to be avoided) and tension ("overloading" your muscles during exercise and thus improving them), you will be less prone to strains caused by picking up something that is too heavy. Regular stretching will also make your muscles more flexible and, therefore, less susceptible to strains.

▶▶ better health

By using weights you can strengthen your joints and increase your bone density, which can help protect you from osteoporosis (brittle bones) later in life.

how to use this book

No matter what you hope to achieve, this book will provide a training schedule for you, regardless of your fitness level.

chapter one: how fit are you?

Shows you how to assess your current fitness level and helps you get started. By looking at your current fitness level, you are much more likely to start training at the right level, which in turn will help you to stick to your training.

chapter two: starting out

Has lots of useful background information, from choosing the right shoes to advice on cardiovascular training and nutrition. You'll discover what you should be eating and in what quantities, how to prevent injuries, and more. Although seeing physical results may take some time, positive benefits (such as feeling good about yourself, having more energy, living healthily, decreasing negative stress, and making new friends) are sure to come earlier in the program.

chapter three: the exercises

Begins the real work. With the knowledge acquired from chapter two, you should be ready to move on to the exercises, which are illustrated in clear pictures, so you can visualize them before you start the program. When you do begin, it is good to have a friend or a mirror on hand so you can check your technique and posture as you go along. It is a lot easier to get it right in the beginning than to correct bad habits later on. The exercises are organized according to body part, so you will know exactly what each exercise is doing.

1 starter level 1

This level is for absolute beginners and shows you exercises that use your own body weight. It is ideal for use when traveling, because the exercises in this section can be done anywhere.

2 starter level 2

This level is for people with a basic knowledge of the toning exercises. It introduces light weights into the program for a more effective workout.

3 refresher level

This level is for people who might be getting back into training or people who are already fit through other forms of exercise. It will help you to develop new skills and will increase muscle strength and tone.

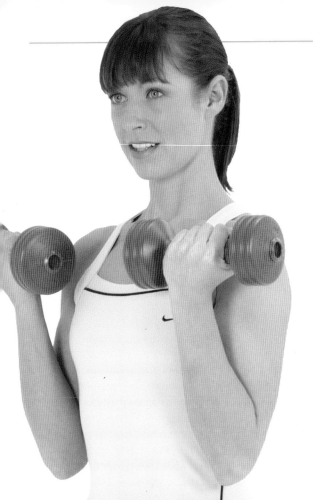

chapter four: the program

Begins the serious training. This chapter sets out a program divided into six levels. If you're new to body toning, you can start at level 1. Those with some toning experience or regular gym users can start (very carefully) at level 3. From level 3 up, advanced programs take you all the way to expert level.

By the time you get to the end of chapter four, you should be confident enough to continue your training in or out of the gym, and you should begin to see some results. So what are we waiting for—let's get going!

4 intermediate level

This level uses a range of equipment and weights so you can start challenging and toning your body.

5 advanced level

This level uses heavier weights to start sculpting and defining your body.

6 expert level

The most advanced phase of the program gives you the knowledge to keep up a challenging, motivating workout for the rest of your life. You should have learned sufficient skills to keep up your interest and avoid boredom.

fitness levels

A low-impact form of exercise like toning is a good place to start increasing fitness and muscle strength. Remember to increase any physical activity slowly and gradually to avoid unnecessary injury.

PHYSICAL ACTIVITY READINESS QUESTIONNAIRE

1 Has your doctor ever said that you have a heart condition and that you should only engage in physical activity recommended by your doctor?

2 Do you feel pain in your chest when you engage in physical activity?

3 In the past month, have you had chest pain when you have not been engaging in physical activity?

4 Do you ever lose your balance because of dizziness or lose consciousness?

5 Do you have a bone or joint problem that could be made worse by a change in your physical activity?

6 Is your doctor currently prescribing drugs for your blood pressure or heart condition?

7 Do you know of any other reason why you should not engage in physical activity?

If you have any "Yes" answers then consult your doctor or relevant specialist.
If you have any other concerns about your fitness it is always best to ask your doctor for a fitness checkup before you start a new training program.

do not start training:

■ If you are not feeling well because of a temporary illness such as a cold. If you have symptoms or signs of illness (such as fever, extreme tiredness, muscle aches, or swollen lymph glands), then rest for at least two weeks before you start training.

■ If you are pregnant, or think you may be pregnant. Take your doctor's advice before making any major changes in lifestyle or activity.

health checks

The questionnaire on the left is a standard document called a PAR-Q (Physical Activity Readiness Questionnaire). It is an easy way to see if it is appropriate for you to start training or if you should consult a doctor first. If you are older than 69 and have been inactive for some time it is a good idea to have a health check with your doctor before you start a training program. If you honestly answer "No" to all the questions, you are fine to start training. If you have any "Yes" answers, then consult your doctor or relevant specialist regarding your intentions and take his or her advice.

how fit are you?

Most people think they are fitter than they are. *Physical Activity and Health: A Report of the Surgeon General Executive Summary* in the U.S. says:

- 60 percent of adults do not regularly follow any exercise program.
- 25 percent of adults do no exercise at all.
- 50 percent of youths between the ages of 12–21 are not active on a regular basis.
- Only 15 percent of adults engage regularly, three times a week, for at least 20 minutes, in vigorous exercise.

CALCULATING YOUR ACTIVITY LEVEL

Calculate your activity level by multiplying your scores for each of the categories listed below. Your activity level is frequency x duration x intensity.

FREQUENCY	SCORE
Less than once a month	1
Few times a month	2
1–2 times a week	3
3–5 times a week	4
Daily or almost daily	5

DURATION	SCORE
Less than 10 minutes	1
10–20 minutes	2
20–30 minutes	3
More than 30 minutes	4

INTENSITY	SCORE
Almost no increase in breathing level, such as golf	1
Slight increase in breathing level, such as baseball	2
Moderately high breathing levels, such as swimming	3
Periodic high breathing levels, such as racket sports	4
Sustained high breathing levels	5

PUTTING THE FIGURES TOGETHER

SCORE	FITNESS LEVEL	COMMENT
Less than 20	Very Low	Sedentary
20–40	Low	Inactive
40–60	Fair	Healthy
60–80	Good	Active
80–100	High	Very active

ready to train?

Start all new training gradually, even if you are generally fit. Any new form of exercise, such as toning, will employ different muscles to those that you would normally use. So start slowly.

Listen to your body, and if you feel like you need to rest, or if you feel an exercise isn't right for you, don't do it or seek advice to check that your technique is correct.

If everything is right, you should be ready to continue.

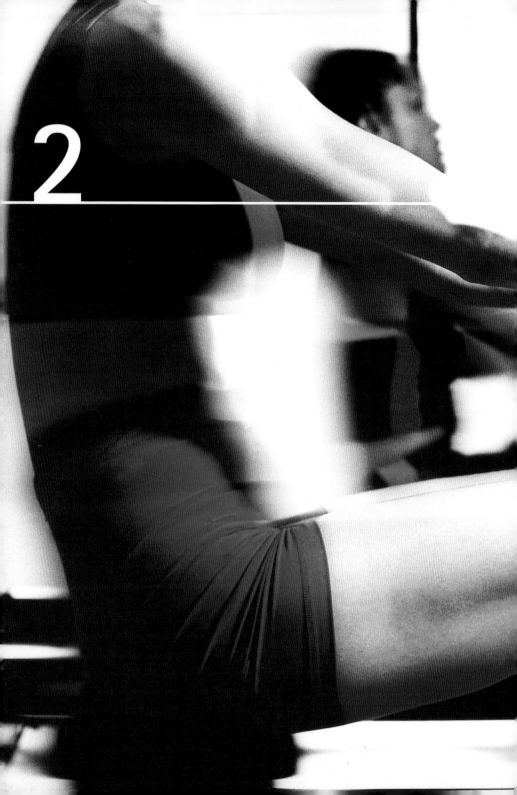

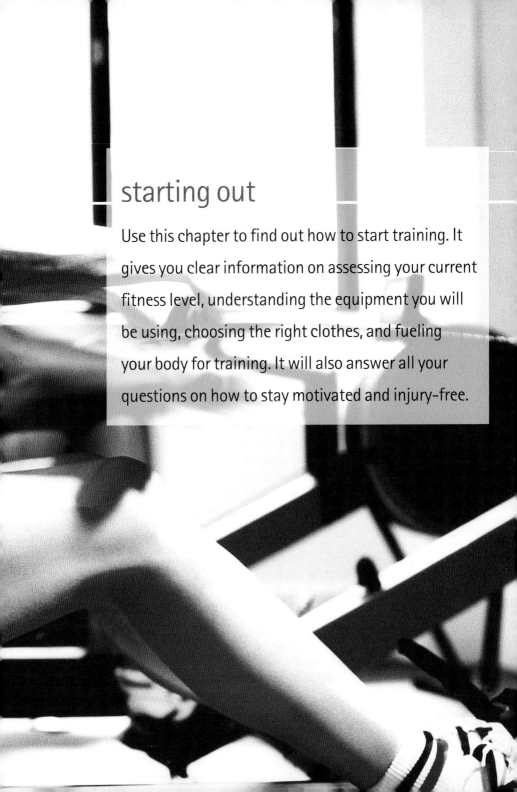

starting out

Use this chapter to find out how to start training. It gives you clear information on assessing your current fitness level, understanding the equipment you will be using, choosing the right clothes, and fueling your body for training. It will also answer all your questions on how to stay motivated and injury-free.

what is fitness?

The term *fitness* can be used to describe your physical, mental, nutritional, emotional, social, or spiritual state. Lack of fitness in one of these aspects can affect the others. To achieve optimal quality of life we should aim to be fit in all areas; this is known as "total fitness" or "total wellness." So a fit person should be able to cope with a high level of cardiovascular (CV) and muscular activity, cope with the stresses of everyday life, and form and maintain relationships. There are several factors affecting physical fitness.

genetic makeup and body type

Your genetic makeup will, to some extent, influence how your body responds when it is trained in different ways.

This is compounded by the three basic body types that will also affect your fitness. Ectomorphs are lean, slim people and tend to be good at endurance events. Endomorphs are more rounded and tend to do well in events requiring all-around ability. Mesomorphs build muscle easily and are generally good at sports involving jumping, throwing, and sprinting.

PHYSICAL FITNESS

There are five components that make up physical fitness:

CARDIOVASCULAR FITNESS	The ability to take in, transport, and use oxygen in the body.
MUSCULAR STRENGTH	The maximum force a muscle can generate against resistance.
MUSCULAR ENDURANCE	The ability of a muscle to exert less than maximum force against resistance over a period of time.
FLEXIBILITY	The maximum range of movement possible around a joint.
SKILL-RELATED FITNESS	Is the possession of certain skills, such as balance, coordination, agility, speed, or reaction time.

No one type of exercise will improve all five areas of fitness, which is why it is important to cross-train—that is to say, you must combine different types of exercise to improve your overall physical fitness. For example, running or cycling will improve cardiovascular fitness, weight training will improve muscular strength and endurance, yoga will enhance flexibility, and a dance class will improve coordination.

age
You tend to become less physically capable as you get older. However, being more physically active can slow down the natural aging process.

lifestyle
Factors such as smoking, drinking alcohol, taking recreational drugs, being stressed, and not getting enough sleep can all affect your fitness level.

diet
You need to eat healthy food to sustain your body in physical activity (see pp. 26–29).

health
Injuries, a cold or other illness, or conditions such as hayfever and asthma can all affect your physical fitness. As we have seen, if you have signs and symptoms of illness—such as fever, extreme tiredness, muscle aches, or swollen lymph glands—then you should rest for at least two weeks before you resume training. Seek qualified medical advice on the issues of asthma and hayfever.

cardiovascular training
Toning and sculpting will help with muscular strength and endurance, motor fitness, and flexibility, but it will not improve your cardiovascular fitness (see pp. 18–19). It is, therefore, important to include CV training with the exercises in this book if you are to achieve total physical fitness.

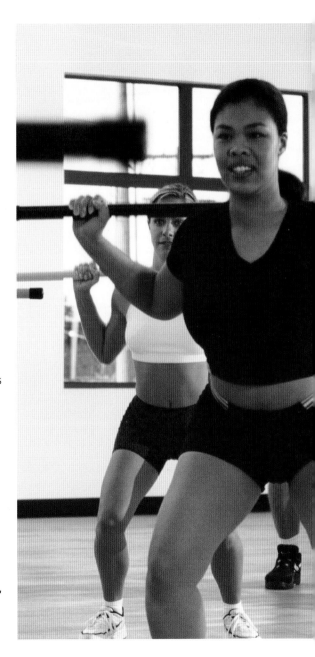

what is CV?

Cardiovascular fitness is often referred to as "stamina," "aerobic fitness," or "endurance." It is your ability to take in, transport, and use oxygen in the body. *Cardiovascular exercise* is defined as any activity that is rhythmic in nature and continuous and uses large muscle groups over an extended period of time. It can be running, rowing, cycling, swimming, or a studio class like aerobics or step.

active muscles

Toning and sculpting will define and strengthen your body. It will also help you burn calories and develop more lean muscles, which will boost your fat-burning potential. Active muscle burns three times more calories than any other body constituent. For optimum fat burning and great body shape you should combine both toning and CV elements in your training.

heart rate

The easiest way to judge how hard you are working is to measure your heart rate. To do this, you first need to determine your resting heart rate.

Find your pulse in your wrist or neck first thing after you wake up. Count how many times it beats in 10 seconds and multiply the answer by six to find out your resting heart rate in beats per minute (bpm).

The average adult has a resting heart rate of 60–80 bpm; this figure will be lower if you are fit and higher if you are unfit.

You then need to determine your maximum heart rate, which is the number of times it is possible for your heart to beat in one minute. This can be estimated by making the following calculation:

220 – your age = age–adjusted maximum heart rate.

Obviously this is an estimate and it is more accurate to have a maximal stress test in a gym, either on a treadmill or exercise bike, to find out your exact maximum heart rate.

It is very hard to measure your heart rate manually when you are exercising. However, lots of cardiovascular exercise machines have an electronic heart-rate monitor built into them, or you can buy a heart-rate monitor, which measures the number of times the heart beats in one minute using electrodes that sense the heart's electrical changes.

making improvements

To improve your cardiovascular fitness, your muscles have to be "overloaded"—made to work at a higher level than they would usually—to make them get stronger. That means that you must train for longer periods of time or at a faster pace. However, never try to improve both at once.

To get the most out of your training, mix in some cardiovascular training with your toning program. Rowing is an excellent CV exercise.

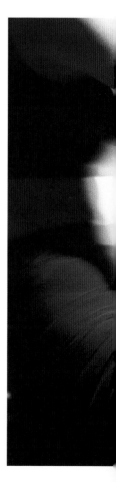

gradual improvement

Don't rush CV training—build up slowly to improve your fitness and avoid injury. As you become fitter, your body will become more efficient, so to burn more calories each day you must either train for longer or exercise at a faster pace. However, you should never increase the intensity and the duration of your workouts at the same time. For example, if you row for 45 minutes each day at a steady pace (6.5 min/mile or 2.10 min/500 m) you will burn about 600 calories. Row at this intensity and duration every day for a week and you will have burned 4,200 calories. Attempting to increase the duration or intensity will only exhaust you.

THE BENEFITS OF CARDIOVASCULAR TRAINING

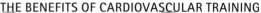

weight loss or weight control

If you burn as many calories as you eat, you will stay the same weight. If you eat more calories than you need, then the excess will be stored as fat around the body. If you can use more calories than you have eaten, then the rest will be taken from the stored fat around the body, and you will lose body fat. To lose 1 lb (455 g) of fat in a week you need to create a deficit of 3,500 kcals (500 kcals per day); this is best achieved with a combination of diet and cardiovascular training.

more efficient lungs

Your lungs do not get bigger as you train, but they do take in more oxygen to be used around the body. The respiratory muscles get stronger so they can work aerobically for longer periods of time or at higher intensities.

improved blood flow

You will have more red blood cells, which carry oxygen around the body, and you will have more blood pumped by the heart around the body. This creates more capillaries to transport the blood to the body, so that there are more avenues for the blood to flow down, which could lower blood pressure.

greater endurance

Your muscles can work for longer as they are getting more blood and oxygen.

lower cholesterol levels

You will have less fat in your blood. Too much saturated fat can lead to high cholesterol levels.

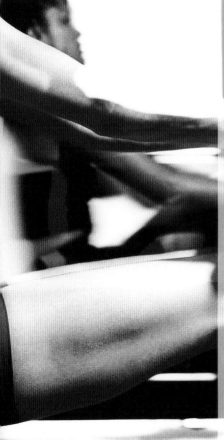

equipment for home training

If you want to train at home, it is not essential to have any equipment, because you can use your own body weight to perform the basic toning exercises (see chapter three). However, as you get stronger you may want to invest in some basic equipment to give yourself a more challenging workout. Most department stores, sports stores, and home-shopping catalogs now have a sports section, so it shouldn't be too hard to find what you need.

Hand weights, barbells, resistance bands, core stability balls (also known as Swiss balls), and body bars are all featured in this book. Once you know the basics, you can create your own program so that you can work as hard as you want, wherever you want, when you want.

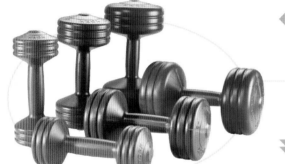

◀◀ hand weights

Hand weights are an important addition to your equipment. They come in a large variety of shapes, sizes, and weights. You can also improvise hand weights by filling plastic bottles with sand or water, though the grip is not as comfortable.

▼ barbell

A barbell is a useful piece of equipment for toning exercises, because you can vary the amount of weight on the bar. As you get stronger, you can add more plates so that you work harder.

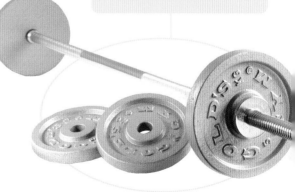

RECOMMENDED WEIGHTS

Choose weights that allow you to complete the recommended sets but leave your muscles tiring toward the end.

A light weight
Is one that you can easily lift, and that becomes tiring only after lots of repetitions (up to 25 reps).

A medium weight
Is one that you can lift for up to 10–15 reps. The last reps should feel difficult.

A heavy weight
Is one that you can only just lift for the required number of times, requiring real effort (6–10 reps).

resistance bands ▶▶

If you do not have much space for storage or training, or are traveling, resistance bands, or dynabands, are perfect. They are tough bands of stretchy rubber that come in different thickness to vary resistance. There are lots of exercises using dynabands for your arms and legs that are just as effective as using weights.

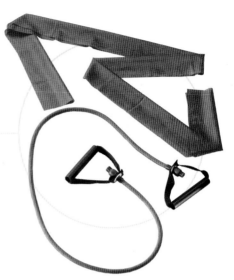

◀◀ core stability ball

A core stability ball, or Swiss ball, challenges your deep abdominal muscles. It can also improve your posture and help strengthen your lower back. Balls come in different sizes. The ball is the right size if, when you sit on it, your legs are bent at 90 degrees. Do not use a stability ball unsupervised if you have high blood pressure or a bad back or are pregnant.

body bar ▶▶

A body bar is a weighted bar, and it is versatile for training arms and legs. It is harder to have bad technique with a bar because it automatically keeps your shoulders and hands in line.

finding the right gym

Most towns now have a gym, and all of them should be happy to let you watch a class or have a look around before you decide to join. When deciding which one to join, ask yourself the following questions:

■ Can I afford it?
■ Is it easy for me to reach, and can I park the car there?
■ Is it clean throughout?
■ Is there a wide range of equipment and classes for me to try?

■ Are the staff friendly and happy to give advice and answer questions?
■ Does it have a day nursery?
■ Does it have women-only facilities? (Some women can feel intimidated in male-oriented environments.)

where to train

There are pros and cons to training at home or in a gym, but it is ultimately a question of where you feel most comfortable and where you can train the most efficiently.

WHERE DO YOU TRAIN?

advantages of training in a gym

■ A good gym will have a wide range of up-to-date equipment, so you should never get bored.
■ There will be expert advice on hand if you have questions about technique or need new ideas.
■ You may be more motivated to train for a solid hour with no distractions if you have made the effort to leave the house.
■ You will meet new people with whom to train.
■ You are more likely to try different types of exercise—for example, aerobics or swimming.

disadvantages of training in a gym

■ It can be expensive.
■ It can be intimidating, especially if you are self-conscious about your appearance or fitness.
■ The equipment can, at first glance, appear confusing. If you have too many choices, you might not know where to start.
■ It is easy to make excuses. You can adopt the "I'll go tomorrow" attitude.
■ Child care or parking may be a problem.
■ It may be too far out of the way from work or home.
■ It may be overcrowded, so that you have to wait for equipment to become available.

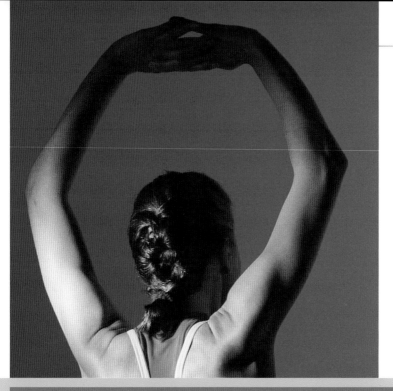

advantages of training at home

- ■ You can train anytime, with a video or at your own pace.
- ■ You don't have to travel anywhere.
- ■ You can often look after your children at the same time.
- ■ There are no subscription fees.
- ■ You don't have to feel self-conscious.
- ■ You don't have to share equipment.

disadvantages of training at home

- ■ There are lots of possible distractions, such as children crying, to telephones ringing, to domestic chores.
- ■ It can be hard to keep motivated for a whole hour.
- ■ There is no one to let you know if you are doing something incorrectly or ineffectively. It is hard to maintain good technique without mirrors.
- ■ It may get boring doing the same exercises on a limited amount of equipment.
- ■ Space might be limited, making it difficult or dangerous to train near the coffee table or television, for example.

looking the part

The main thing when choosing your sports clothing is to find something comfortable to wear. Old baggy T-shirts, shorts, and sweatpants are fine (despite the range of expensive clothing often on display in gyms), and they ensure you have enough room for a full range of movement.

SHOES

The most important thing you can invest in for training is your footwear. Good sports shoes will help protect your knees, ankles, shins, and hips by absorbing some of the impact of jumping or running, for example. It is impossible to train well if your feet are hurting, so a pair of well-fitting, supportive shoes is essential.

Choose sports shoes that are designed for athletics rather than aesthetics. Get advice from the sales assistant in the store to check which shoes are most suitable for the exercise you will be doing.

CHOOSING THE RIGHT FOOTWEAR

1 Look for footwear specifically designed for the exercise you are doing. For example, running shoes are different to tennis shoes. Cross-training shoes are suitable for the body-toning exercises in this book.

2 Try on both shoes (everyone has one larger foot) to make sure you have the right size; your feet should feel supported, not cramped.

3 Walk around the store to see if they feel comfortable. Jump up and down, and see how they feel when you land so you can get an idea of how they would feel during exercise. Be aware of any parts of your foot that feel like they would rub or blister after training.

4 Be guided by comfort and suitability, not by price.

5 Old shoes lose their stability, so change your training shoes every 6 to 12 months to help prevent unnecessary injury.

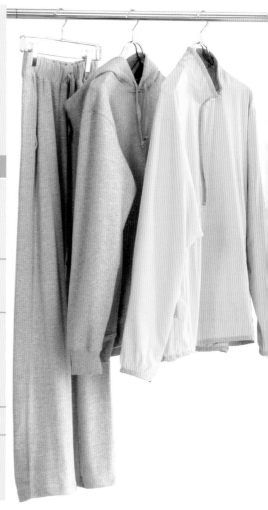

CRITICAL SUPPORT

Women undertaking any nonstationary exercise must invest in a good sports bra, regardless of bust size. A sports bra supports and protects the breasts more than a regular bra.

LOOKING GOOD

Although you can wear almost anything, if you are having trouble getting motivated, it is sometimes a good idea to go out and buy a new gym outfit. For some people, if they look the part they feel the part. It is a commitment to getting started.

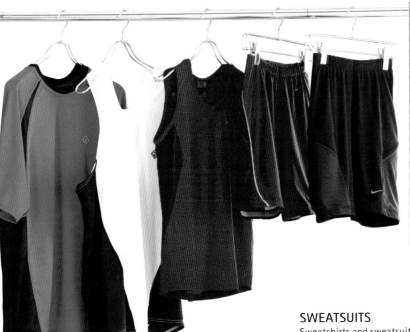

If you are training in a public place, consider other people. Make sure your gym kit is clean, because it is very unpleasant to be overpowered by the next person's body odor. And tiny shorts with no underwear are not always attractive to other gym users!

SWEATSUITS

Sweatshirts and sweatsuits are often comfortable and are especially good for training in cold rooms because they help you to feel warmer, quicker. However, take care, because your muscles may not be as warm as your body feels, and they will still need to be stretched properly before exercise.

STATE-OF-THE-ART FABRICS

T-shirts can be bought in various "wicking" materials, which claim to keep the sweat away from your body, keeping you more comfortable as you train. These fabrics have been championed by many top athletes, but it is up to you to decide if they work for you.

exercise nutrition 2

to lose weight
If you want to lose weight you need to expend more calories than you take in. You should aim to cut your caloric intake by no more than 500 calories a day, which would mean you would lose 1 lb (455 g) a week.

wonder diets

There are always lots of new diets advertised in newspapers, books, and magazines, each claiming that it will make you lose fat fast. These designer diets all work on the principle that most people are looking for a miracle solution that will help them lose fat without having to exercise or change their lifestyle.

starvation mode

Be suspicious of diets that encourage you to remove one of the basic food groups from your diet; you need a

ENERGY BALANCE EQUATION

- When output is greater than input you lose weight

- When output is less than input you gain weight

- When output is equal to input your weight stays the same

balanced diet for good health. Be particularly wary, too, of diets that encourage you to halve your caloric intake to around 1,000 calories a day, or less. By severely cutting your calories,

MANAGING YOUR CALORIC INTAKE

It is best to control weight loss by combining a healthy diet with regular exercise. Your body needs food and calories even when it is resting, but the amount of food you need in a day depends on several things (these figures are approximate, because everyone's metabolism is different and everyone expends a different amount of calories while doing the same things):

SEX (basal rate)
Men—11 calories per pound (24 calories per kilogram) of body weight.
Women—10 calories per pound (22 calories per kilogram) of body weight.

LIFESTYLE
Add an additional 30 to 40 percent for a sedentary job, such as office work.
Add an additional 50 to 60 percent for an active job, such as construction work.

EXERCISE
Add 400 calories per hour of steady exercise (for example, jogging on a treadmill)
Add 600 calories per hour of vigorous exercise (for example, an intensive session on the cross-trainer at the gym)

EXAMPLE
A 130 lb (60 kg) female office worker who exercises steadily for 1 hour per day will need:
130 lb x 10 = 1,300 + (35% x 1,300) = 1,755 + 400 = 2,155 calories per day

you could actually put on weight. Not knowing where the next meal is coming from, your body will go into starvation mode, holding on to the food you eat for as long as possible, and your metabolic rate (the speed at which you digest and process food) will lower. When you start to eat normally again, any fats or carbohydrates will be expended even more slowly, which is why people often end up bigger than they were before they started dieting. If you are continually going on crash diets, research has shown that it can take up to a year of training for your metabolism to start working normally.

EATING MORE HEALTHILY

1 Always eat a good breakfast that will keep hunger at bay and give you plenty of energy. For example two whole-wheat biscuits (to fill you up) with a banana (for instant energy), or whole-wheat toast (to fill you up) and jam for instant energy).

2 Take healthy snacks to work with you so you don't get hungry and tired. Eat fruit, low-fat yogurt, or nuts and raisins. If you don't let your energy stores drop, you will be less likely to reach for a coffee or a chocolate bar to give you a quick energy boost.

3 Eat more at lunchtime than at dinnertime, when you are more likely to spend time in front of the TV. You will expend more calories during the day and you will store more food in the evening when you are sedentary.

4 Try to eat more complex carbohydrates, because these take longer to digest and will leave you feeling full for longer. Try switching to whole-grain foods.

5 Cut down on alcohol. A large glass of beer has the same number of calories as a chocolate bar.

6 Eat smaller portions, and beware of low-fat processed foods. People are always tempted to eat larger portions of food labeled "low fat" because they think it is healthier. However, many low-fat foods contain more additives, because fat acts as a preservative, and many are high in salt. In some cases it is better to eat less of the regular version than more of the low-fat alternative. It is also true that if you deprive yourself of certain foods—chocolate, for example—you are more likely to crave them. So enjoy the occasional piece of chocolate; just don't eat the whole bar.

7 Drink more water. Sometimes hunger is actually an indication of thirst.

8 Try to eat more unsaturated fats that are liquid at room temperature, such as olive oil, because they will boost your immune system and help to lower the levels of saturated fats in your blood that cause high cholesterol levels and heart disease.

9 By eating more healthily you should have more energy, recover from illness and injury more quickly, and lead a longer life.

developing correct posture

Good posture will make you look and feel more confident. It will also make you look thinner and taller, and it will decrease the risk of lower-back pain. Research has shown that lower-back pain is a major physical limitation in people's lives, and it is often used as an excuse not to exercise, which can lead to further muscular weakness and deconditioning. It is also one of the main reasons for absence at work in the Western world. Try to think about your posture not only in these exercises but also in your everyday life—for example, when sitting at a desk or carrying a heavy shopping bag.

Achieving good posture takes time, so don't feel discouraged if you sometimes forget to stand or sit properly. Persevere and good posture will eventually become the norm.

what is good posture?

The spine contains around 33 vertebrae.
- There are seven vertebrae in the cervical area; The first vertebra, called the atlas, forms a pivot joint with the second vertebra, which allows you to turn your head from side to side.
- The thoracic area has 12 vertebrae, which form joints with your ribs to protect your internal organs from injury.
- The five lumbar vertebrae in the lower back are the largest and strongest bones of the spine.
- The five sacral vertebrae are fused and allow no movement.
- The four coccygeal vertebrae are also fused and form the coccyx.

natural curves

A normal spine is designed to form an S shape, which centers the head over the body. It has four natural curves. The S shape provides shock absorption, which prevents you from hurting yourself when you jump up and down or move suddenly.

Between the vertebrae are intervertebral disks that act as shock absorbers. When individuals have correct posture, the vertebrae in the spine sit on top of one another naturally. We start to feel pain if the disks become damaged or nerves get trapped in the vertebrae because of bad posture or repeated unsafe movements.

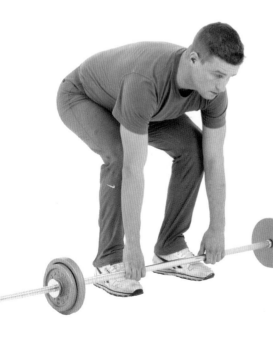

ACHIEVING GOOD POSTURE

Remember
If you are suffering
from back pain,
consult a qualified
medical practitioner.

Stand up tall in front of a mirror

1 Round your shoulders all the way forward, then squeeze them all the way back. Now bring your shoulders to a central position so your chest feels open and your shoulder blades feel pulled down toward your spine.

2 Keep your shoulders in position and push your tummy out as far as you can, as if you are pretending to be pregnant, then suck your tummy all the way in. Breathe out so you can feel your tummy muscles working, but still breathe easily. Imagine you are wearing a belt and you have it on the middle hole so that it is neither really loose nor so tight it hurts.

3 Tilt your pelvis forward as if you are scooping your buttocks underneath you, then push your pelvis all the way back so you have to arch your back. Settle halfway between the two. Imagine your hips are like a bucket of water that can swing forward or back; you are aiming to get the water in the bucket level in the middle.

A natural position

You should be able to breathe easily, and you should feel light, tall, and relaxed. Try to remember how this feels as you move onto the basic exercises, and try to practice it every day by correcting yourself every time you notice yourself sitting or standing with poor posture. Over time it will become your natural posture.

preventing injuries

The most significant benefit of exercising can be felt in your day-to-day life. Training on a treadmill will enable you to run for the bus, keep up with your children, and walk up escalators without getting out of breath. Lifting weights will strengthen your muscles so that you can carry more shopping bags or move heavy items without injury.

lifting technique

You should try to remember the techniques learned in the gym to avoid injuries in everyday life. Back injuries are both common and troublesome, but they can often be avoided by improving your posture and lifting technique. Sudden jerky movements are particularly dangerous when lifting heavy objects at home and in the workplace.

Bend your knees to lift something heavy. Try to keep a straight back with your abdominal muscles ("abs") contracted. Come up slowly in a smooth movement, through a basic squat position, with most of your body weight over your heels. Keep the heavy item you are lifting close to your body. If it is too heavy to lift safely, don't lift it. If you have any injury, seek medical help before attempting any exercise program.

COMMON COMPLAINTS

ankles

Twisted and strained ankles usually come from walking on uneven surfaces or from wearing heeled or platform-soled shoes, in which you can't feel the floor properly. Take extra care when walking up or down stairs, especially if you are in a hurry, and look out for any wet patches of sweat or spilled water in gyms. Strengthen ankles by doing calf raises (see p. 52).

shin splints

Shin splints are a common and painful repetitive injury that occur when the shin bone starts separating from the shin muscle. They are caused by any movement, such as running or jumping, that requires you to put your heels down. They can also be caused by running with the wrong shoes, running on hard surfaces, and overtraining the legs with activities that require pounding or rapid and hard foot movement. When you are running, try to run with a heel-to-toe action, and if you are jumping, always land through the whole foot. Rest is really the only cure for shin splints, though you should consult a sports medicine practitioner if it is really severe.

THE R.I.C.E APPROACH TO INJURIES

R—rest
Stop training until the injury has cleared up, and try to keep your weight off the damaged area.

I—ice
Firmly apply an ice pack or a bag of frozen peas wrapped in a towel. Alternatively, rub the injured area with an ice cube for 15 minutes every hour, or as often as you can manage.

C—compression
Bandage the area firmly (but not so that it restricts the circulation) to reduce inflammation. Anti-inflammatory drugs can also help.

E—elevation
Raise the injury to reduce the blood flow in the early stages, thereby minimizing tissue damage.

FITNESS AVOIDS INJURY

By generally being stronger, fitter, and more active you are less likely to get injured because you are more coordinated and more aware of your body. Improved flexibility might save you a strained hamstring if you slip on ice in the winter, because your muscles are more elastic and more able to cope with sudden movements.

Similarly, by strengthening your core muscles you are less likely to fall over if you are standing on a bus or train that stops suddenly, because you are able to control yourself better. By being more aware of how your body is supposed to work, you also become better at predicting when something is about to cause you injury. Fitter people move in a more controlled manner and should suffer fewer injuries and major ailments in old age.

knee strains

Knees are usually injured by bad alignment. You should always aim to have your knees in line with your ankles, directly over your middle toes. Women tend to suffer knee problems more than men because their hips are wider, which means their thigh bone automatically makes a triangle shape to the knee joint. To get your knees to fall in a straight line if you're a woman often takes a lot of practice, especially if you have proportionately wide hips. Bad technique in squats and lunges or wearing high heels for long periods can also cause knee pain.

blisters

Blisters are a common complaint. If you are doing a lot of running or high-impact activity, they are difficult to avoid completely. The most common cause of blisters is ill-fitting shoes, closely followed by old or thin socks. You should also tie your shoelaces; untied laces do not secure your shoes to your feet properly, and the resulting friction will cause blisters.

sticking to it

Before you start to learn the basic toning exercises, it is good to know what you hope to achieve. There is no instant fitness regimen that will make you an athlete or shrink you to the size of a runway model overnight. It is important to start your training program slowly and safely, and to build up gradually. When people go from doing no activity to training vigorously every day, they usually get injured or bored and give up.

try something new

Thankfully, there is such a wide variety of exercises available today that it is possible for everybody to find something that is enjoyable.

Most gyms offer a wide choice of classes, from hip-hop and salsa dancing, to kickboxing, step, and more traditional aerobics sessions. Going to a class is a great way to make new friends and arranging to meet someone at a gym is a good way to make sure you go. Give new things a try; you don't have to go back if you don't enjoy yourself.

making exercise fit

Find a gym or a routine that fits into your life. There is no point joining a gym a long way from your home because it will be too easy for you not to go. You should also be realistic about your goals.

TRAIN SMART

Try to train SMART. This means that your goals should be:	**ACHIEVABLE** "At the moment I can complete two sets of 10 push-ups with a 30-second break."
SPECIFIC "I want to complete 20 push-ups without stopping."	**REALISTIC** "Completing 20 push-ups without stopping is the next step from what I can currently do."
MEASURABLE "That's 20 push-ups, not somewhere between 15 or 25."	**TIME ORIENTED** "I want to achieve this within 1 month."

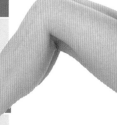

USEFUL GOAL IDEAS

Set yourself one aim at a time. For example, "I am going to concentrate on losing body fat" or "I am going to tone my shoulder muscles."

Write your goals down somewhere you will see them every day, like a note on your fridge or computer screen.

Have a fitness goal, such as being able to run for 2 miles (3 km) in 20 minutes.

Think positively, believe that you can achieve greater fitness, and remind yourself of the benefits of training, such as better muscle tone or cardiovascular fitness, when you are losing motivation.

Focus on positive ideas. Instead of thinking, "I'm getting tired," think, "I can really feel this working."

Get a friend or family member to remind you to do your exercises.

OVERCOMING COMMON BARRIERS

1 I have children to look after.

Join a gym with a day nursery, or follow an exercise video at home while your children are sleeping. Walk them to school instead of driving. Go roller blading, swimming, or cycling with your children.

2 I sometimes have to work late.

Go for a run or join a gym and train at lunchtime or before work if you know you will not have time in the evening.

3 I can't afford to join a gym.

Go for a walk or a run or do some exercise at home.

4 I get bored easily.

Keep changing your routine. It is perfect for overall fitness to do lots of different things, such as swimming, dancing, weight training, yoga, and running.

5 I need to rest in my spare time.

If you start exercising and leading a more healthy lifestyle, you will find that you have more energy.

6 I feel too shy to exercise at the gym.

Exercise at home where you can't be seen by anyone else. When you feel more confident, think about going to a gym with a friend or relative.

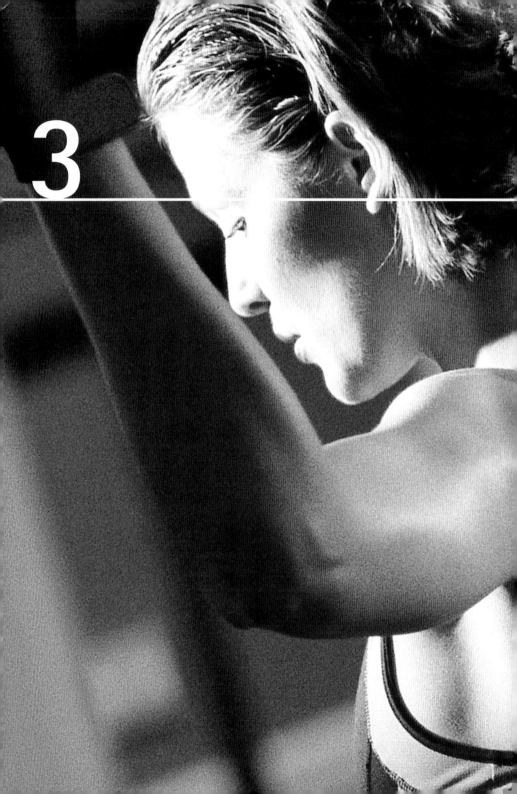

3

the exercises

In this chapter you will see all the exercises demonstrated with correct technique. It is important to learn how to perform the exercises safely and effectively before you start adding weights. It is worth taking the time to check your technique in a mirror to make sure it is the same as the one illustrated in the pictures. It is easier to learn exercises properly at the start than to develop bad habits and then have to change them. Start practicing the exercises with no equipment; later, you can add resistance or core stability tools.

warm-up ideas 1

It is important to warm up before attempting any form of exercise. A warm-up is basically a rehearsal for the workout ahead. It helps you to facilitate skillful and coordinated movements, such as small squats, leg curls, knee lifts, and bicep curls, which will be developed in the main workout.

mobility exercises

Mobility exercises should be performed on all the joints so that the whole body is prepared for a workout. They should be started as small movements that get bigger, until you are using your full range of movement after a few repetitions.

ANKLE MOBILITY

1 Heel digs—Alternate right and left leg, bending your supporting leg and digging your heel out in front of you. Repeat 10–20 times.

2 Toe taps—Repeat the movement as above but tapping your toe out in front of you. Repeat 10–20 times.

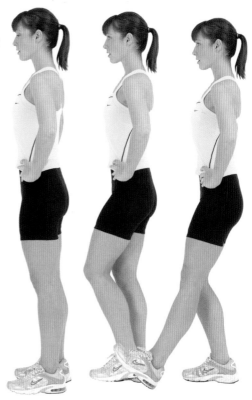

THE 1, 2, 3 OF A WARM-UP

A warm-up should consist of three components:

1 Mobility exercises—To increase body temperature and to release the shock-absorbing and lubricating synovial fluid in the joints.

2 Pulse-raising exercises—To gradually increase the heart rate and pump more blood, oxygen, and nutrients through the muscles before the hard exercise starts.

3 Short stretches—To prepare the large muscle groups that will be used in the proposed activity.

HIP MOBILITY

1 Pelvic tilts—Tilt your pelvis forward and back four times with your knees slightly bent.

2 Hip circles—Tilt your hips forward, to the right, to the back then to the left, keeping your tummy in and knees slightly bent. Repeat four times in one direction, then four times in the other.

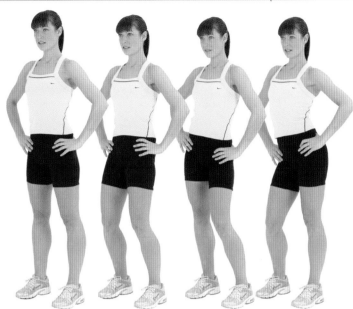

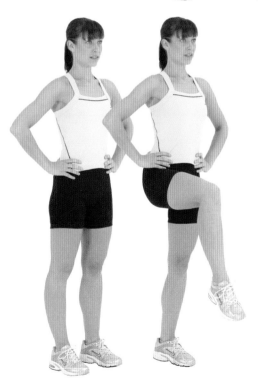

KNEE MOBILITY

Knee lifts—Stand with correct posture (see pp. 30–31). Alternate right and left legs, lifting your knee to hip height. Keep the supporting leg slightly bent. Repeat 20 times.

CLICKING JOINTS

If you hear a clicking sound from your joints, don't worry unless the sound is accompanied by pain. If you feel pain, consult a sports medicine practitioner.

warm-up ideas 2

NECK MOBILITY
CERVICAL VERTEBRAE
With good posture, look right and left under control, keeping your eye level the same. Repeat 4–6 times. Then look forward and, while keeping your shoulders still, tilt your ear toward your shoulder in a smooth movement then back to center. Repeat to the other side 4–6 times.

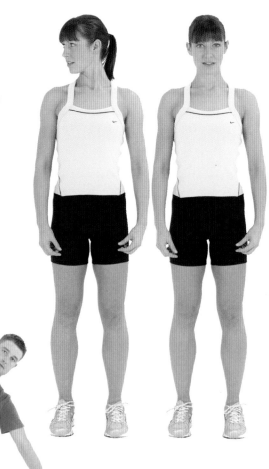

LOWER–BACK MOBILITY
LUMBAR VERTEBRAE
Side bends—Stand with your feet hip-width apart, toes pointing forward and knees slightly bent. Without tipping forward or backward, reach to the floor on your right side then back up to center. Repeat to the left. Alternate sides 6–10 times.

SHOULDER-GIRDLE MOBILITY

Shoulder rolls—Stand with upright posture and abs in. Draw the shoulders up toward the ears, then gently roll the shoulders back and down 4–8 times then reverse the movement 4–8 times, lifting the shoulders up then rolling forward.

MIDDLE-BACK MOBILITY
THORACIC VERTEBRAE

Side twists—Stand with knees slightly bent, feet hip-width apart, tummy in. With your hands to the side of your head, turn your body to the back of the room, keeping your head in line with your spine. Return to the front of the room under control, then twist to the other side. Avoid twisting the knees. Repeat 4–8 times.

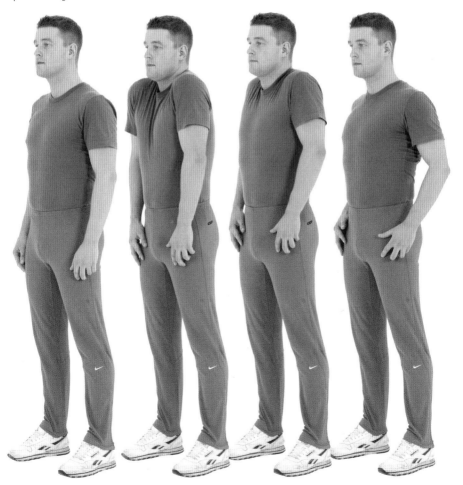

pulse-raising exercises

Pulse-raising exercises should increase the heart rate gradually over a period of a few minutes.

You should be aiming to work at 50–60 percent of your maximum heart rate. A good way to judge this is by imagining your breathing to be at level zero if you were lying down totally still. At the other end of the scale, level 10 would be when you were running so hard that you were gasping for breath.

You should aim to train at level 5 or 6, where you are aware of your breathing and are starting to feel hot.

CALF RAISES (SEE P. 52)

With good posture, push up onto the balls of your feet then come back down. Accompany this by raising your arms so they are straight above your head. Lower your arms as you lower your heels. Do 20 repetitions. Ignore the arm element to this exercise if it affects your balance.

KNEE LIFTS
(WITH ALTERNATE HAND TO KNEE)

Try to stand upright and don't slouch your back. Aim to lift your knees to hip height. Alternate right hand to left knee and vice versa. Do 15–20 repetitions.

Level	
10	Gasping for breath
9	Struggling to breathe
8	Running fast
7	Breathing deeply
6	Starting to sweat and getting out of breath
5	Running faster
4	Jogging gently
3	Starting to hear your breath
2	Walking quickly
1	Walking slowly
0	Lying still

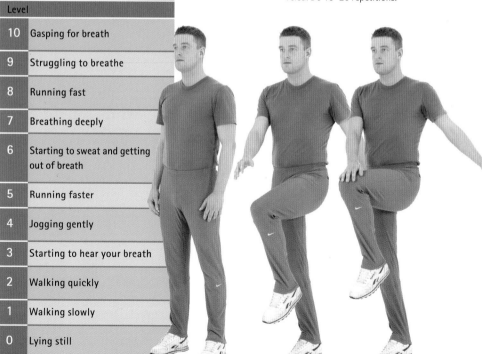

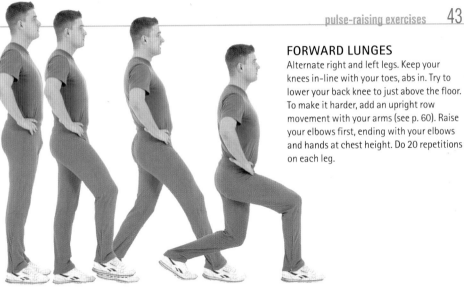

FORWARD LUNGES

Alternate right and left legs. Keep your knees in-line with your toes, abs in. Try to lower your back knee to just above the floor. To make it harder, add an upright row movement with your arms (see p. 60). Raise your elbows first, ending with your elbows and hands at chest height. Do 20 repetitions on each leg.

LEG (HAMSTRING) CURLS

Adopt an upright posture and bend your knees (with your knees in-line with your toes). Move from the knee, curling your ankle toward your buttocks. Do 20 repetitions on each side.

SMALL SQUATS

Stand with your knees in line with your toes, your feet hip-width apart, and your abs in. Sit back like you are going to sit down on a chair, then come back up. Do 20 repetitions.

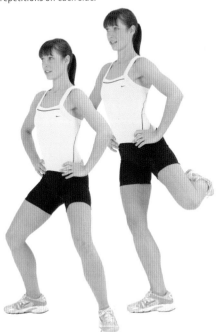

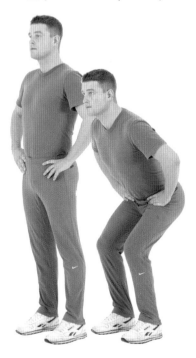

preworkout stretches 1

There is no scientific evidence that says that you have to stretch before a workout, but it is a good idea to prepare your body as fully as possible before you start training; this is especially true if you are starting a new type of exercise. Stretching increases the blood flow to the muscles, which makes muscle strains less likely.

When your muscles are cold they are tight and can easily be pulled when you try to use them. But when warm, they bend and stretch and are much more pliable.

The following preparatory stretches are for your whole body and can be done in any order. They will prepare your body for the rigors of a workout but are not intended to increase your flexibility significantly. You therefore have to hold each position for 10 seconds.

Remember to do right and left sides, and pay attention to your posture. Try to find your balance by keeping your eyes fixed on something still and holding in your tummy. If you are wobbly, you can hold onto a wall for greater control and stability until you get used to the positions. Try to move in and out of each position slowly. You may find it useful to have a mirror to check that you are in the same position as the person in the picture.

THE STRETCHES

The scientific names for the muscles are included in case you come across them in reference books or articles. Don't let them confuse you, though, because you don't need to remember Latin names to stretch effectively.

HIP FLEXOR STRETCH

Bend both legs, moving one forward, and raise the heel of your back leg. Scoop your pelvis under and push it forward to feel a stretch in the hip flexor of your back leg.

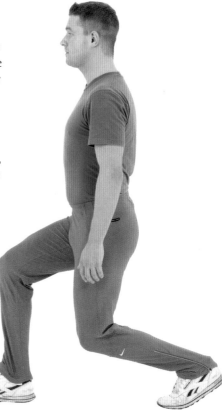

BACK STRETCH
(TRAPEZIUS AND POSTERIOR DELTOID)
Round your shoulders forward as if you are
hugging a big beach ball, keeping your
tummy in.

CHEST STRETCH
(PECTORALS)
Place your hands on your buttocks or clasp
them behind your back and lift them away
from your buttocks. Bend your elbows and
squeeze them together, stretching out the
chest. This exercise can also be added to a
calf stretch.

CALF STRETCH
(GASTROCNEMIUS STRETCH)
Bend your front knee and keep your back
knee straight. Position your toes pointing
forward and your knees in-line with your
toes. Lean your body weight forward, and
imagine a straight line from your head to
your back heel. You should feel the stretch
in the calf of the leg that is set back.
You can add on a stretch for your upper
back by interlocking your fingers and
pushing your hands forward.

SIDE STRETCH
(LATISSIMUS DORSI AND OBLIQUES)
Start with your feet hip-width apart and
your knees slightly bent. Reach up, then
lean to the side with one arm stretched
over your head so that it feels as if you are
lifting up and out of your hips rather than
just bending to the side. Try not to lean
forward or backward.

preworkout stretches 2

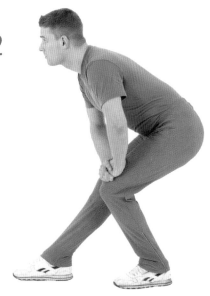

HAMSTRING STRETCH
(BACK OF LEG)
Bend your back leg with the foot flat on the floor and place your front leg straight out in front, foot flat on the floor. Try to keep your back straight, and think about pulling your shoulder blades together to open out the chest and flatten your back. Keep your head in-line with your spine, and check that your knees are in line with your toes. To increase the stretch, think about lifting your buttocks higher. You should feel the stretch in the back of your front leg.

INSIDE-THIGH STRETCH
(ADDUCTOR)
Stand with your knees bent and pointing outward in-line with your toes. Bend down and use your elbows to increase the stretch by pushing your knees out. Don't let your buttocks drop down lower than your knees. Be careful to make sure that your knees do not roll in and that they are in line with your middle toe.

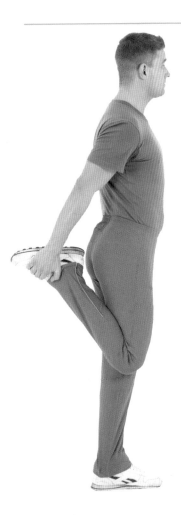

FRONT-THIGH STRETCH
(QUADRICEPS)

Stand on one leg with your supporting knee slightly bent, abs in. Keep your hips pointing forward as you bring your heel to your buttocks, holding the front of your ankle. If you are wobbly, hold on to a wall, hold your tummy in, fix your eyes on one point, or hold your ear to stabilize you. Don't worry if you feel strange holding your ear; it does work.

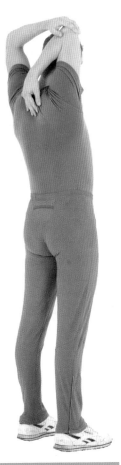

REAR-ARM STRETCH
(TRICEPS)

1 With good posture, push your arm straight up in the air, then bend at the elbow so that your hand drops down to the back of your neck.

2 Increase the stretch by gently pulling on the back of the arm with your other hand. Try to keep a gap between your chin and your chest so your head is in line with your spine.

You should now feel ready to start some basic toning exercises. If you are feeling cold, repeat a few of the pulse-raising exercises until you feel warm again. Alternatively, gently jog in place.

BASIC TONING EXERCISES ▶▶ ▶▶

The following exercises can be done in any order, but it is best to start with the largest muscle groups because smaller muscles get tired quicker than larger ones.

leg-toning exercises 1

NARROW SQUATS
BUTTOCKS AND THIGHS (GLUTES AND QUADRICEPS)
Stand with your feet positioned hip-width apart; knees, ankles, and feet in-line; and abs in. Stick your buttocks out and back, as if you are going to sit on a chair. Think about squeezing your buttocks as you straighten your legs to come up. You may find it easier to balance with your arms out in front of you. Make sure that your knees aren't bent forward and that your calves are at a 90-degree angle to the floor; this is so you don't put pressure on your lower knee. Most knee injuries sustained at the gym come from squatting with bad technique.

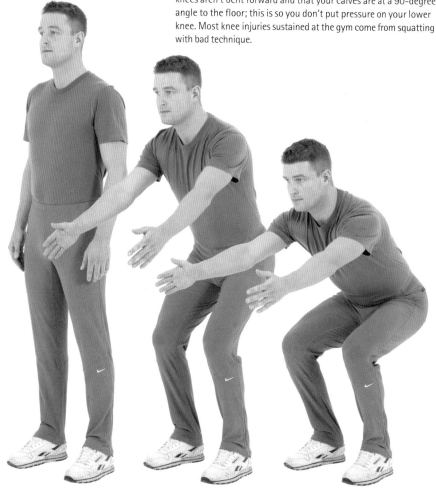

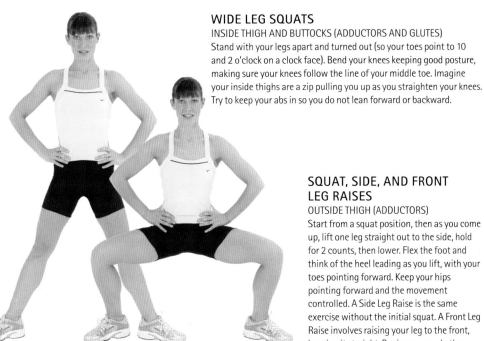

WIDE LEG SQUATS
INSIDE THIGH AND BUTTOCKS (ADDUCTORS AND GLUTES)

Stand with your legs apart and turned out (so your toes point to 10 and 2 o'clock on a clock face). Bend your knees keeping good posture, making sure your knees follow the line of your middle toe. Imagine your inside thighs are a zip pulling you up as you straighten your knees. Try to keep your abs in so you do not lean forward or backward.

SQUAT, SIDE, AND FRONT LEG RAISES
OUTSIDE THIGH (ADDUCTORS)

Start from a squat position, then as you come up, lift one leg straight out to the side, hold for 2 counts, then lower. Flex the foot and think of the heel leading as you lift, with your toes pointing forward. Keep your hips pointing forward and the movement controlled. A Side Leg Raise is the same exercise without the initial squat. A Front Leg Raise involves raising your leg to the front, keeping it straight. Beginners can do the Front Leg Raise lying on the floor.

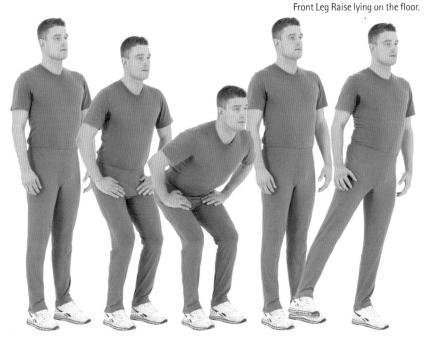

leg-toning exercises 2

STATIC AND STEP-FORWARD LUNGES

HIP FLEXOR AND BACK OF THIGH (ILIOPSOAS AND HAMSTRINGS)

Stand in a squat position and take a large step back with one leg. Keep your back leg on the ball of the foot all the time as you lower the knee toward the floor; don't let it touch the floor before moving it back up. Check that your toes are pointing forward and your knees are following the line of your feet. You are aiming to form a right angle on both legs in the lower position. Make sure you are not bending your front knee forward and your calf stays vertical to protect your knees; keep your abs in, and maintain good posture. If you feel wobbly, move your legs farther apart to provide a more stable base. A Step Forward Lunge involves taking a large step forward with one leg, rather than backward. All the rest of the exercise remains the same.

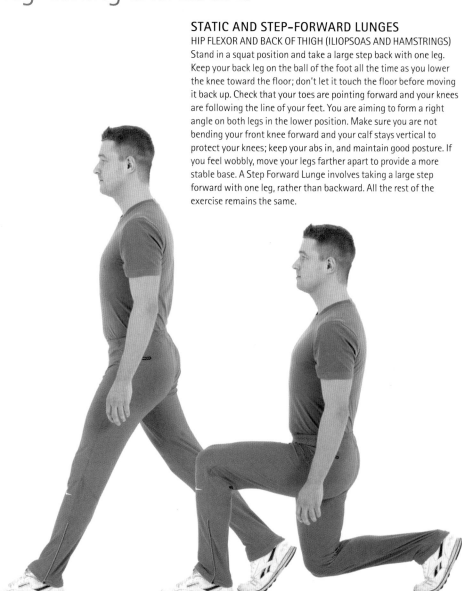

SQUATS WITH BARBELL—ADVANCED TECHNIQUE
Stand with your feet shoulder-width apart and the barbell across your shoulders. Bend your knees, keeping your back straight, until your thighs are no more than parallel with the floor. Push back up to standing.

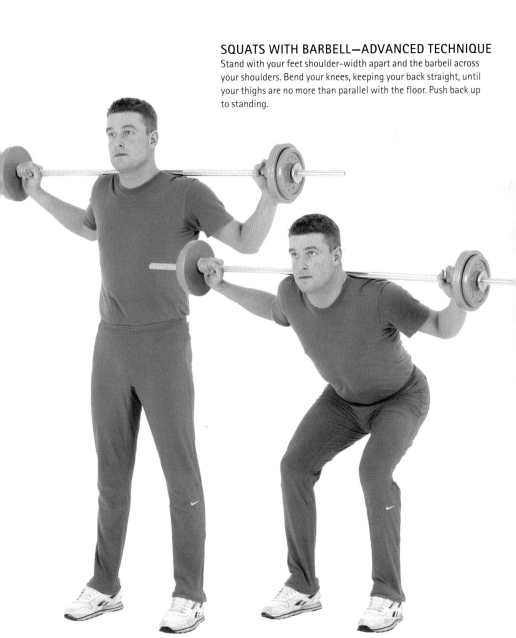

leg-toning exercises 3

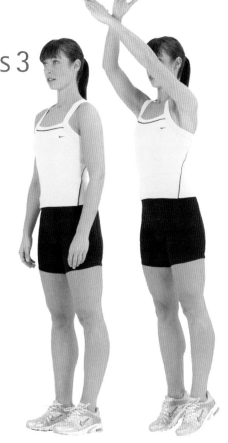

CALF RAISES
CALVES AND BACKS OF YOUR LEGS
(GASTROCNEMIUS AND SOLEUS)
Position your feet hip-width apart, keep your ankles
in-line with your toes as you come up on the balls of
your feet, pause, then lower your heels. Stand tall
with your buttocks and abs in. This is a good
exercise to do in queues or waiting for the bus.

LYING BRIDGE
BUTTOCKS, ABS, AND BACKS OF LEGS (GLUTES AND HAMSTRINGS)
Lie on the floor with your legs bent, hip-width apart, with your feet flat on the floor. Push
your hips up in a straight line from your neck to your knees. Keep your neck relaxed on the
floor. Squeeze your buttocks and hold the position. You can raise and straighten one leg at a
time to make the exercise harder.

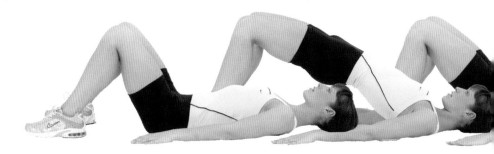

DEAD LIFT WITH BARBELL
QUADRICEPS, HAMSTRINGS, GLUTEUS MAXIMUS,
AND ERECTOR SPINAE

Stand with your feet shoulder-width apart, toes
underneath the bar. Bend your knees, making sure that
your knees, ankles, and toes are in-line. Stand up, pushing
up from your knees and leading with your shoulders,
keeping the barbell close to your body. Lower the bar with
control. You can also use hand weights for this exercise.

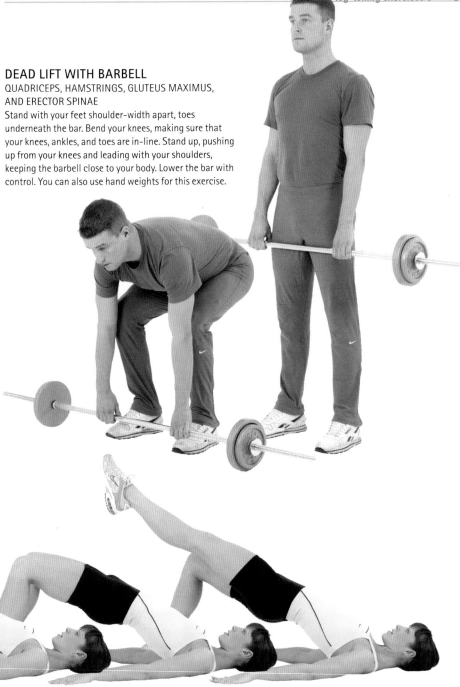

abdominal-toning exercises 1

SIT-UPS
UPPER ABS (RECTUS ABDOMINUS)
Lie on the floor with your knees bent, hip-width apart, and your feet flat on the floor. Think about pulling your tummy in as you do when standing with correct posture. With control, lift your head and shoulders off the floor, keeping your tummy pulled in as you come up, then lower. Breathe out on the way up, breathe in on the way down. Keep looking at the ceiling and imagine you have a tennis ball between your chin and your chest; this will keep your head in-line with your spine. Slide your hands over your thighs to your knees as you come up, then return them to your hips. To make it harder (as shown below), hold your hands by your ears with your elbows wide.

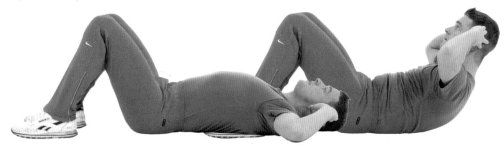

SIT-UPS ON CORE STABILITY BALL—ADVANCED TECHNIQUE
Lie on the ball with your legs bent at 90 degrees. Taking care to balance properly, use your abdominals to lift your head and shoulders up, while looking at the ceiling.

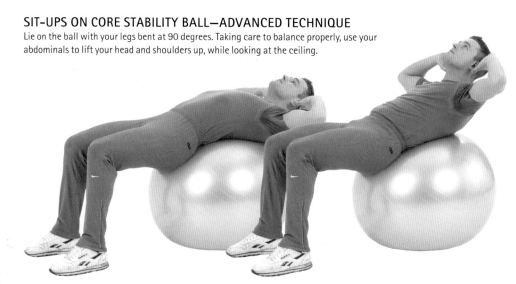

OBLIQUE CURLS
UPPER SIDE ABS (INTERNAL AND EXTERNAL OBLIQUES)
Position yourself for a sit-up, with your hands by your ears and your elbows wide. Move your body up, then twist to one side but keep looking at the ceiling. Come back to a sit-up position and gently lower your head back to the floor. Try to use your tummy muscles to move your body rather than just your elbows. Maintain a consistent gap between your chin and your chest.

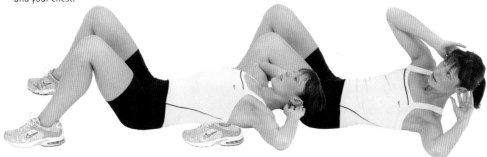

OBLIQUE REACHES ON CORE STABILITY BALL—ADVANCED TECHNIQUE
Lie on the ball with your legs bent at 90 degrees. Stretch your arms out to the side, palms facing up. Keeping your legs still, turn your upper body to the left. Come back to center, then repeat on the other side.

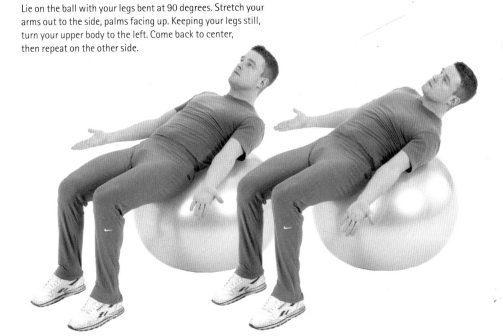

abdominal-toning exercises 2

LEG RAISES
LOWER ABDOMINALS
Lie flat on the floor with your knees bent up and your feet flat on
the floor, hip-width apart. Slowly lift your legs into the air until
your feet are above your hips (keeping your legs bent as they were
at the starting position) then lower under control. Pull your tummy
muscles in to support your lower back as you raise and lower your
legs. If your lower back hurts, try raising one leg at a time until
you feel stronger.

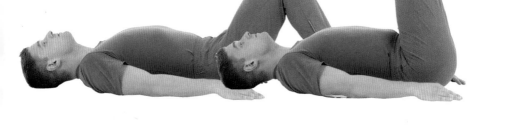

LEG RAISES USING CORE STABILITY BALL—
ADVANCED TECHNIQUE
Lie on your back with your arms by your sides and your feet flat on the
floor. Gripping the ball between your legs with your feet, breathe out
and lift your legs over your hips. Use your abdominals to lift your legs.

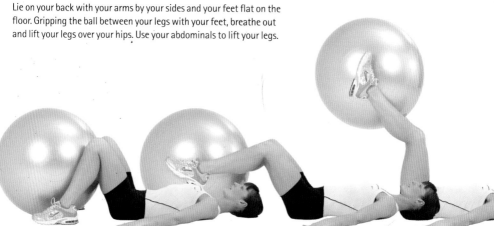

RAINBOWS
LOWER OBLIQUES

Lie on the floor with your legs bent in the air. Slowly drop your legs to one side so your knees almost touch the floor, then come back up to center and repeat to the other side. Keep the movement smooth and continuous. It should feel like you are drawing an rainbow shape with your feet. Bend your knees to make the exercise easier. If you are a beginner, keep both feet on the floor, and drop your knees to either side.

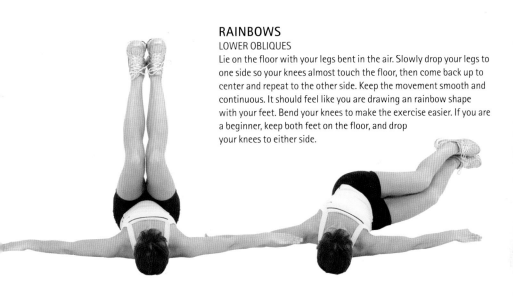

REVERSE CURLS
LOWER ABDOMINALS

Lie flat on the floor. Have your legs slightly bent in the air, above your hip bones, with your feet flexed. Imagine you are pushing the soles of your feet flat onto the ceiling as you squeeze your tummy inward to lift your buttocks up, then lower.

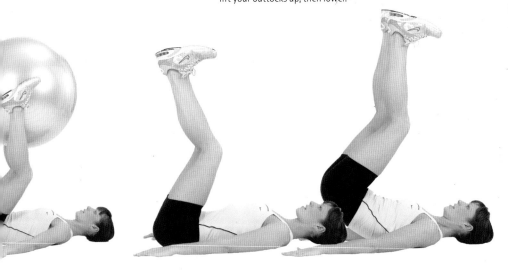

toning the deep abdominal muscles

The following exercises will work the deeper layer of abdominal muscles (also known as the transverse abdominals), which will help you achieve a strong stomach and better posture.

V-SIT
TRANSVERSE ABDOMINALS

Sit up as tall as you can with your knees bent and feet on the floor. Open your chest and place your arms on your shins to start. Lean back, trying to keep your back in a straight line and your tummy in until you are in a V shape. Try to keep breathing and don't lean back any farther as you lift your legs, still bent, off the floor. Move your arms to your sides, without touching the floor. Hold for as long as you can. If you can't lift your legs up, keep them on the floor while sitting in the V shape, holding your tummy in. You will soon build sufficient strength to do the full exercise.

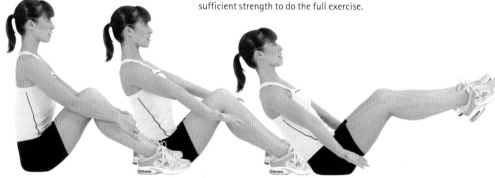

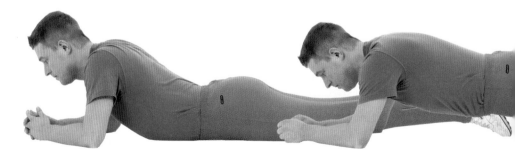

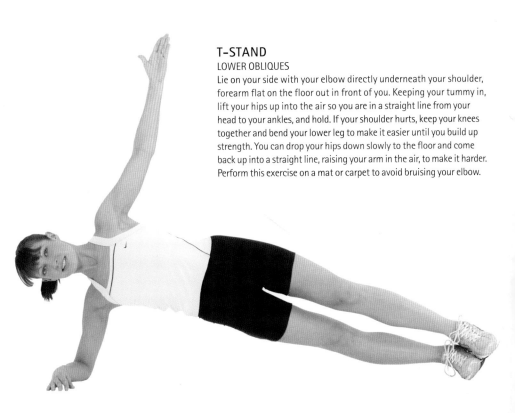

T-STAND
LOWER OBLIQUES

Lie on your side with your elbow directly underneath your shoulder, forearm flat on the floor out in front of you. Keeping your tummy in, lift your hips up into the air so you are in a straight line from your head to your ankles, and hold. If your shoulder hurts, keep your knees together and bend your lower leg to make it easier until you build up strength. You can drop your hips down slowly to the floor and come back up into a straight line, raising your arm in the air, to make it harder. Perform this exercise on a mat or carpet to avoid bruising your elbow.

PLANK
TRANSVERSE ABDOMINALS

Lie on your front with your weight rested on your forearms, and suck in your tummy. You should have a gap between your tummy and the floor. Keep your tummy sucked in as you come up onto the fleshy part of your knee and hold the position. You can stay there or, to make it harder, come up into full plank with your body in a straight line and your weight on your toes. Keep breathing with your abs pulled in as tight as they will go.

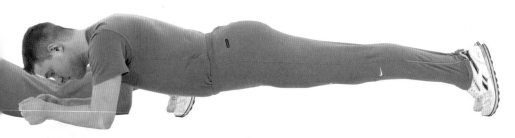

shoulder-toning exercises

SHOULDER PRESS
TO WORK YOUR SHOULDERS
With your feet hip-width apart or with one foot bent back on the ball of the foot, start with the bar by your chest. Have your hands about 6 in. (15 cm) wider than your shoulders and lift the bar above your head, in front of your face, so you don't have to lean back, and return to chest height. Straighten your arms but do not lock out the elbows. Keep the movement smooth and controlled.

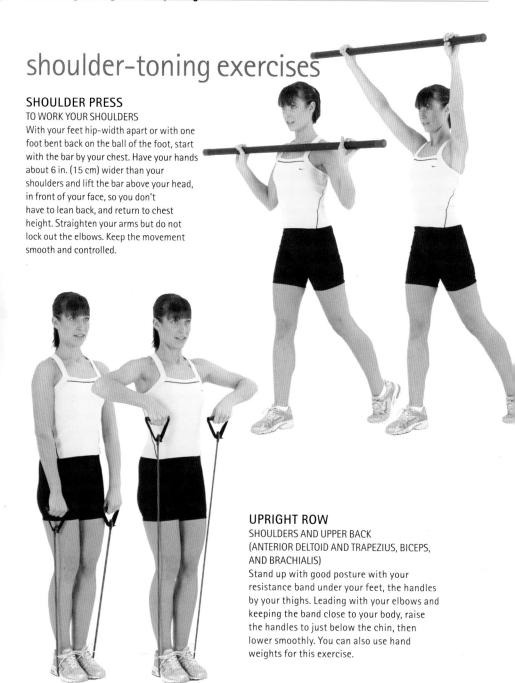

UPRIGHT ROW
SHOULDERS AND UPPER BACK
(ANTERIOR DELTOID AND TRAPEZIUS, BICEPS, AND BRACHIALIS)
Stand up with good posture with your resistance band under your feet, the handles by your thighs. Leading with your elbows and keeping the band close to your body, raise the handles to just below the chin, then lower smoothly. You can also use hand weights for this exercise.

BEHIND NECK PRESS

**UPPER ARMS AND UPPER BACK
(LATISSIMUS DORSI, TRAPEZIUS, BICEPS,
AND BRACHIALIS)**

Hold your resistance band (or body bar) with
your palms facing away from you, about
double-shoulder-width apart, straight up in
the air, but with elbows soft. Lower the
resistance band (or body bar) down behind
your head to lightly touch your shoulders.
Think about your elbows pulling down first,
and then returning your arms slowly back to
the extended position. Remember to keep
your tummy in and your back straight.

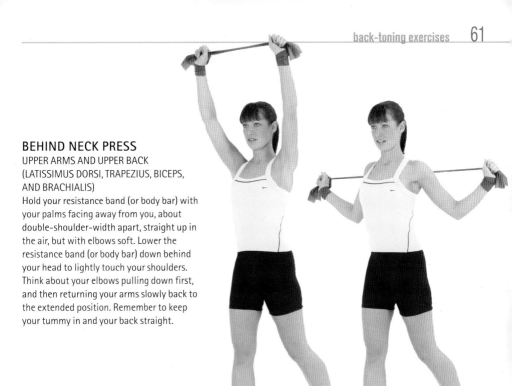

back-toning exercises

Every time you exercise your abdominal muscles, it is important to do some back
extensions to work the opposite muscle group.

PRONE FLY

TRAPEZIUS AND RHOMBOIDS

Come up like a back extension with your
hands by your ears and elbows wide. When
you are lifted up, squeeze your elbows
together toward your spine, come back up to
the starting position,
and lower.

BACK EXTENSIONS (BELOW)

TO STRENGTHEN YOUR LOWER BACK (RECTUS SPINAE)

Lie flat on your tummy and keep your face to the floor to keep your
head in line with your spine. Have your hands on your lower back or
by your ears, with elbows wide. Lift your shoulders off the floor, not
letting the skin on the back of your neck wrinkle, and lower in a
smooth movement. This exercise shouldn't hurt. If it does, then you
are coming up too high.

chest- and bicep-toning exercises

BOX PUSH-UP
(PECTORALS AND TRICEPS)
Come onto your hands and knees with your hands wide, fingers pointing forward, tummy in, and back flat. Bend your elbows and try to get your nose and chest onto the floor and come back up. You are aiming to get your chest onto the floor in between your hands. Try not to let your back arch.

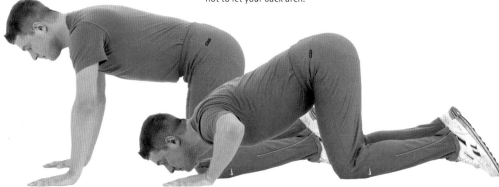

PUSH-UP ON CORE STABILITY BALL—ADVANCED TECHNIQUE
Lie face-down on the ball, your hands and feet on the floor. Walk your hands forward, rolling your legs over the ball. When your knees are on the ball, start your push-ups. The farther your hands are from the ball, the harder the push-up becomes. Be careful to maintain good balance at all times.

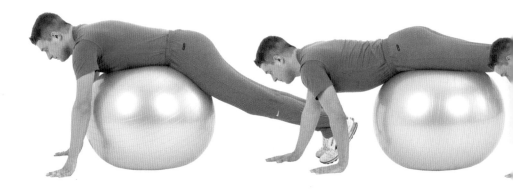

PHASE TWO PUSH-UP
TO MAKE YOUR PUSH-UPS HARDER
From being on your hands and knees, come forward onto the fleshy part of your knee. Keeping your back flat, tummy in, hands wide, and fingers pointing forward; bend your elbows to get your chest and nose onto the floor, then push back up. Your chest should be level with your hands. Keep the movement slow and controlled.

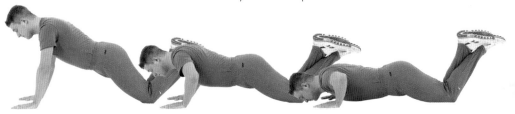

FULL PUSH-UP
Keep the same arm position as above but come up onto the balls of your feet. Bend your elbows, lowering your body to the floor (keeping your back straight and not letting your tummy touch the floor), then push back up under control.

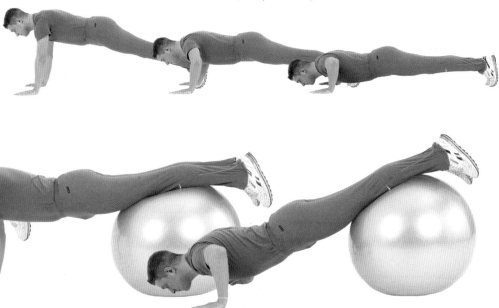

arm-toning exercises

BICEP CURLS
FRONTS OF YOUR ARMS
Stand with good posture, feet hip-width apart, or with one leg bent back on the ball of your foot if you feel your back is arching. Hold the weights by your thighs then bend your elbows, until your hands are level with your shoulders, then slowly lower them. Keep your elbows against the sides of your body and control the movement. You can use hand weights, the barbell, body bar, or resistance band (held under your feet) for this exercise.

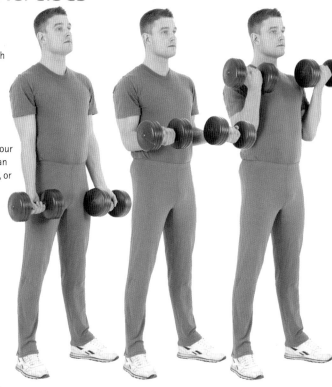

TRICEP DIPS
BACKS OF YOUR ARMS
Sit on the floor with your tummy in and your back in a straight line. Have your hands behind you with your fingers pointing toward your buttocks. Bend your elbows, trying to keep them going behind you, and come up. To make it more difficult, position your hands farther away from your buttocks or lift your buttocks up to use your whole body weight to train your arms.

TRICEP DIPS ON CORE STABILITY BALL— ADVANCED TECHNIQUE

Start with your knees bent and your palms face-down behind you on the ball. Lower yourself from your shoulders, bending your arms, then push back up. To make the exercise harder, straighten your legs. Keep good balance throughout the exercise.

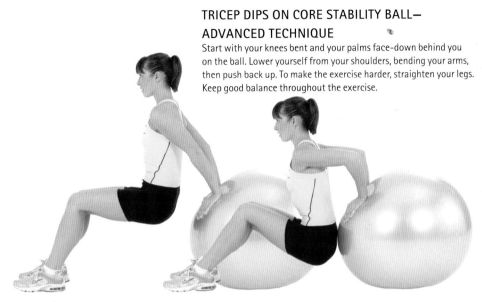

LATERAL AND FRONT RAISES

UPPER ARMS AND FRONT OF SHOULDER (MEDIAL DELTOID)

Stand with good posture and your knees soft. Start with the dumbbells against the sides of your thighs, palms facing inward. Raise the dumbbells to the side, to shoulder height. Lead with the elbows and avoid locking them out. Try to keep a smooth continuous, controlled movement. You can also lift your arms to the front. This is called a Front Raise.

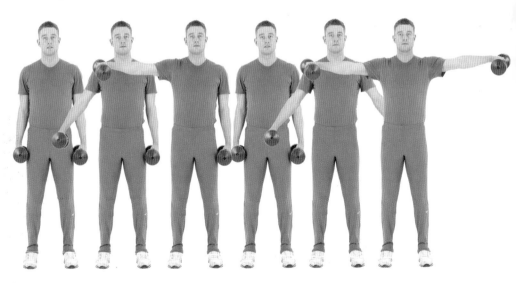

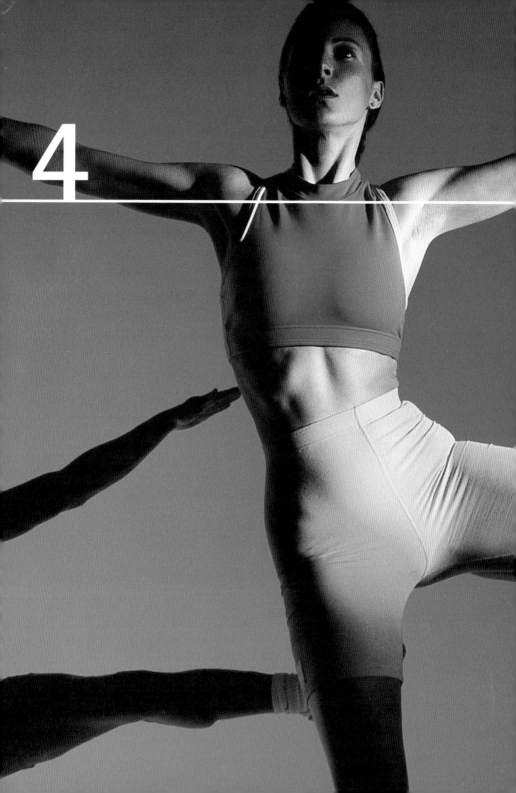

4

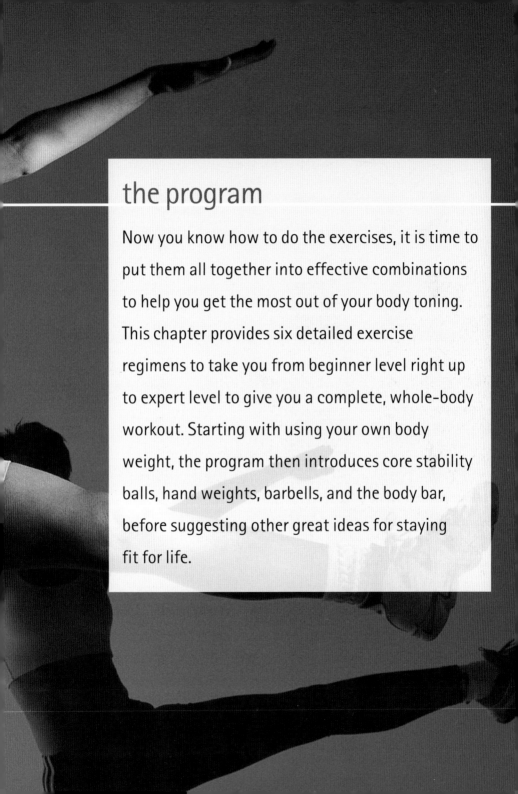

the program

Now you know how to do the exercises, it is time to put them all together into effective combinations to help you get the most out of your body toning. This chapter provides six detailed exercise regimens to take you from beginner level right up to expert level to give you a complete, whole-body workout. Starting with using your own body weight, the program then introduces core stability balls, hand weights, barbells, and the body bar, before suggesting other great ideas for staying fit for life.

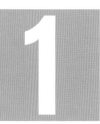

using your own body weight

A new start is all about taking small steps to achieve your goals. Even if you are fit, it is advisable to take a couple of days to familiarize yourself with the basic exercises in this program. You must also make sure you are training with correct technique. Any new form of exercise uses different muscles, so it is worth building up slowly to avoid any unnecessary pain or injury. Don't be in a rush to skip to level 4 immediately. If these exercises feel easy, try to slow them up, performing every movement in a slow, controlled manner and trying to use your full range of movement so that you bend down or straighten up as far as you can. If you find that you are fit or naturally strong in an area, move on to level 2 after a few days rather than a week.

check your technique
Refer to chapter three (pp. 36–65) and keep checking your technique as you execute each new exercise. If you have a friend training with you, he or she can check your technique; otherwise you will need to use a mirror. Look at yourself from all angles in the mirror to make sure you aren't getting a false impression; a squat, for example, can look fine from the front, whereas from the side you may notice your knees bending forward.

basic equipment
You can do level 1 exercises anywhere, because they use your own body

RECOMMENDED PROGRAM

exercise pace
When following the program, the speed with which each exercise should be completed is given in "counts." All counts are single counts unless otherwise stated.

MONDAY	A block (hips, legs, buttocks, and core muscles)
TUESDAY	Rest day
WEDNESDAY	B block (abs, arms, shoulders, chest, and back)
THURSDAY	Rest day
FRIDAY	A block
SATURDAY	Rest day
SUNDAY	B block

weight and don't need any equipment. For floor exercises, it is recommended that you invest in a fitness mat, because a wooden floor can easily bruise your spine and carpet can burn your skin. If you don't have a mat, try using a towel or folded sheet instead.

getting started

The exercises are divided up into blocks. The A block concentrates on your hips, legs, buttocks, and core muscles, and the B block works mainly your abdominals, arms, shoulders, chest, and back. Alternate the A and B blocks, as shown in the recommended program opposite (p. 68).

BEFORE YOU START

If you miss a day, try to do both the A and B blocks on the next day. Try not to train for 4 days in a row, because you will be exhausted for the rest of the week. You should also avoid doing the same block on consecutive days, because your muscles will need time to recover. Each block should take you about 20 minutes. Don't rush through the exercises—make each one count.

WARM-UP

Before you start each day, warm up for 10–15 minutes. Follow the exercises on pp. 38–47 or have a brisk walk, do some skipping, or perform some small squats and lunges to prepare your muscles for the workout to come. Remember to stretch out your muscles, paying particular attention to the ones used in your block for that day.

program 1 ▶▶

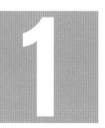

using your own body weight (cont.)

A BLOCK
If you have trouble keeping your balance, try holding on to the back of a chair. Also remember to maintain good posture and pull in your abdominals. This will help aid stability as you do your exercises.

SQUAT/LUNGE COMBINATION

1 10 x narrow squats

2 10 x right-leg-back static lunges

3 10 x narrow squats (2 counts down, 2 counts up)

4 10 x left-leg-back static lunges

5 4 x narrow squats (4 counts down, 4 counts up)

WIDE-LEG-SQUAT/CALF-RAISE COMBINATION

1 10 x wide leg squats

2 5 x quick calf raises, hands on hips or on a chair

3 5 x calf raises (2 counts up, 2 counts down)

4 10 x wide leg squats (2 counts down, 2 counts up)

5 5 x repeat calf raises (2 counts up, 2 counts down)

SIDE LEG RAISES

10 x side leg raises to the right
10 x repeat to the left

FRONT LEG RAISES
Lie on your back, left knee bent, foot flat on the floor, right leg straight

1 10 x front leg raises, right leg, toes pointed
10 x repeat on left leg

2 10 x front leg raises, right leg, flexed foot
10 x repeat on left leg

LYING BRIDGE

Hold for 30 seconds, rest then repeat.

THE PLANK

Hold for 30 seconds, rest then repeat.

T-STAND

Top leg raised 6 in. (15 cm), foot flexed. Hold for 30 seconds, rest then repeat. Repeat on the other side.

V-SIT

Keeping feet flat on the floor, hold for 30 seconds.
Rest then repeat.

Stretch out your muscles, paying particular attention to your legs and buttocks.

B BLOCK

Start by lying on the floor, knees bent up, feet flat on the floor

LEG RAISES

10 x leg raises, right leg, knee bent
10 x repeat on left leg

RAINBOWS

10 x alternate to the right and left (keeping your feet on the floor)

SIT-UP/TRICEP-DIP COMBINATION

1 10 x sit-ups, sliding your hands from your thighs to your knees
10 x tricep dips, buttocks on the floor

2 10 x sit-ups (2 counts up, 2 counts down)
10 x tricep dips (2 counts down, 2 counts up)

OBLIQUE-CURL/SIT-UP COMBINATION

1 10 x oblique curls (alternate right then left)

2 5 x sit-ups (4 counts up, 4 counts down)

3 10 x repeat oblique curls

4 5 x sit-ups

REVERSE CURLS

Hold the reverse curl position, holding your abs in for 30 seconds, rest then repeat.

BACK EXTENSIONS

20 x back extensions, hands on your lower back or on the floor bent in front of you to make it easier.

STANDING PUSH-UP

Perform this exercise facing a wall. For a wide standing push-up, place your hands 6 in. (15 cm) wider than shoulder-width apart. For a narrow standing push-up, place your hands shoulder-width apart.

1 10 x wide standing push-ups
10 x narrow standing push-ups

2 Repeat sequence.

DEAD-LIFT/SHOULDER COMBINATION

1 10 x dead lift (2 counts down, 2 counts up)
10 x behind neck press
10 x repeat dead lift

2 10 x shoulder press
5 x dead lift
10 x behind neck press
5 x repeat dead lift
10 x repeat shoulder press

BICEP-CURL/UPRIGHT-ROW COMBINATION

1 10 x bicep curls
10 x upright row

2 10 x bicep curls (2 counts up, 2 counts down)
10 x upright row (2 counts up, 2 counts down)

LATERAL-RAISE/FRONT-RAISE COMBINATION

1 5 x lateral raise, right arm
5 x repeat on left arm
5 x lateral raise, both arms

2 5 x front raise, right arm
5 x repeat on left arm
5 x front raise, both arms

Stretch out your muscles, paying particular attention to your abdominals, arms, and back.

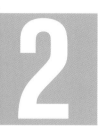

using light weights

Do you feel ready to make the exercises harder? If anything hurts or feels difficult, stay at level 1 for another week for that particular exercise. Check back to chapter three if you need to brush up on your technique for any exercise.

improvisation

You will need some light weights for this part of the program. If you are training at home and do not have equipment, you can use cans of baked beans or small bottles filled with water or sand instead of hand weights. For leg exercises that call for a body bar, you can do double the repetitions to get the

same workout without the bar. Keep the same format as used on level 1, with your A and B blocks, to get a whole-body workout.

warm–up

Before you start each day, remember to warm up for 10–15 minutes, following the exercises suggested on pp. 38–47. Alternatively, have a brisk walk or cycle, and perform some small squats and lunges to prepare the muscles for the workout to come. Arm circles are great for getting the blood flowing around the body. Stretch out your muscles, paying particular attention to the ones used in your block for that day.

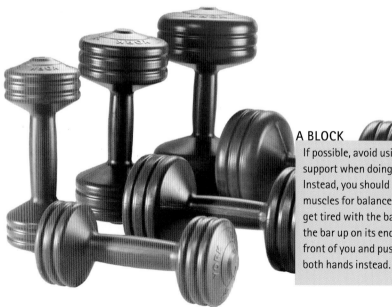

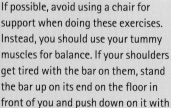

A BLOCK

If possible, avoid using a chair for support when doing these exercises. Instead, you should use your tummy muscles for balance. If your shoulders get tired with the bar on them, stand the bar up on its end on the floor in front of you and push down on it with both hands instead.

SQUAT/LUNGE COMBINATION

All exercises with a light body bar on your shoulders

1 10 x narrow squats

2 10 x right-leg-back static lunges

3 10 x narrow squats (2 counts down, 2 counts up)

4 10 x left-leg-back static lunges

5 4 x narrow squats (4 counts down, 4 counts up)

SIDE LEG RAISES

All exercises with a light body bar on your shoulders, or placed on its end on the floor in front of you

1 10 x side leg raises to the right
10 x repeat to the left

2 5 x side leg raises to the right (2 counts up, 2 counts down)
5 x repeat to the left

FRONT LEG RAISES

Lie down, knees bent, feet flat on the floor

1 10 x front leg raises, right leg, toe pointed. Brush your right foot along the floor until your leg is straight, then lift the leg straight up and down.
10 x repeat on left leg

2 10 x front leg raises, right leg, flexed foot
10 x repeat on left leg

WIDE-LEG-SQUAT/CALF-RAISE COMBINATION

All exercises with a light body bar on your shoulders

1 10 x wide leg squats

2 10 x quick calf raises

3 5 x calf raises (2 counts up, 2 counts down)

4 10 x wide leg squats (2 counts down, 2 counts up)

5 5 x calf raises (2 counts up, 2 counts down)

LYING BRIDGE

1 Hold for 30 seconds.
10 x scoop your buttocks under, then push up until you are in a straight line from neck to knee again.

2 Hold for 30 seconds.
10 x repeat scoop and push up

THE PLANK

Hold for 10 seconds, rest then repeat twice.

T-STAND

With your lower leg bent, push your hips up. Hold for 30 seconds, rest then repeat. Repeat on the other side.

V-SIT

With your feet on tiptoe, lean back into a V, hold for 30 seconds, rest then repeat.

Stretch out your muscles, paying particular attention to your legs and buttocks.

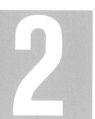

using light weights (cont.)

B BLOCK
Start by lying on the floor, knees bent, feet flat on the floor

LEG RAISES

1 10 x leg raises, keeping the knees bent (alternate right and left)

2 10 x leg raises, both legs
If your lower back starts to hurt, pull your abs in harder or go back to exercising one leg at a time until you are stronger.

RAINBOWS

10 x point your toes and lift your feet 2 in. (5 cm) off the floor. Alternate right and left sides.

SIT-UP/TRICEP-DIP COMBINATION

1 10 x sit-ups, hands by your ears

2 10 x tricep dips, buttocks on the floor, placing your hands farther away from your buttocks than in level 1.

3 10 x sit-ups (2 counts up, 2 counts down)

4 10 x tricep dips (2 counts down, 2 counts up)

OBLIQUE–CURL/SIT–UP COMBINATION

1 10 x oblique curls (alternate right and left)

2 5 x sit-ups (4 counts up, 4 counts down)

3 10 x repeat oblique curls

REVERSE–CURL/SIT–UP COMBINATION

1 5 x reverse curls

2 5 x sit-ups (4 counts up, 4 counts down)

3 Repeat combination.

BACK–EXTENSION/PUSH–UP COMBINATION

1 10 x back extensions, hands by your ears as in a sit-up position

2 10 x wide-arm box push-ups

3 10 x back extensions

4 10 x box push-ups, hands under your shoulders to work your triceps.

how's it going?

Everyone has different natural capabilities. If you feel strong enough to do full push-ups, for example, feel free to do so. Similarly, if you do not feel strong enough to start adding weights, just use your body weight only. The aim is to enjoy a challenging, but safe, workout.

DEAD-LIFT/SHOULDER COMBINATION

All exercises with light hand weights

1 10 x dead lift (2 counts down, 2 counts up)

2 10 x behind neck press

3 5 x dead lift (4 counts down, 4 counts up)

4 10 x shoulder press

5 5 x dead lift (2 counts down, 2 counts up)

6 10 x behind neck press

7 5 x dead lift (4 counts down, 4 counts up)

8 10 x shoulder press

BICEP-CURL/UPRIGHT-ROW COMBINATION

All exercises with light hand weights

1 10 x bicep curls

2 10 x upright row

3 10 x bicep curls (2 counts up, 2 counts down)

4 10 x upright row (2 counts up, 2 counts down)

LATERAL-RAISE/FRONT-RAISE COMBINATION

All exercises with light hand weights

1 5 x lateral raise, right arm

2 5 x repeat on left arm

3 5 x lateral raise, both arms

4 5 x front raise, right arm

5 5 x repeat on left arm

6 5 x front raise, both arms

Stretch out your muscles, paying particular attention to your abdominals, arms, and back.

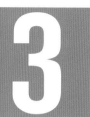

picking up the pace

reviewing your progress

Having come this far—and with two levels of training under your belt—now is a good time to assess your progress and remind yourself of your goals. Have a look back and remember what you wanted to achieve by training. At this stage, you should feel comfortable with the increase in the amount of repetitions and sets, and feel more toned and energized.

avoiding monotony

Exercise should be part of your routine now. However, if you find that going through your program day after day is becoming monotonous, you should mix in an activity (for example swimming, cycling, or running) that will add variety and challenge your body in different ways.

developing at your own pace

Finally, you should listen to your body. If you are ready to move on to level 3, do so, but if you find particular exercises difficult, revert back to level 2 for that part of the program. You could also do an extra set of an exercise you find difficult or check your technique in a mirror to make sure you aren't making any basic mistakes.

RECOMMENDED PROGRAM REMINDER

Before you start, remember your warm-up and stretches.

MONDAY	A block (hips, legs, buttocks, and core muscles)
TUESDAY	Rest day
WEDNESDAY	B block (arms, abs, shoulders, chest, and back)
THURSDAY	Rest day
FRIDAY	A block
SATURDAY	Rest day
SUNDAY	B block

A BLOCK (30-MINUTE WORKOUT)

SQUATS

All exercises with a light body bar on your shoulders

1	10 x narrow squats
2	10 x narrow squats, right heel raised
3	10 x narrow squats, both feet flat on the floor (2 counts down, 2 counts up)
4	10 x narrow squats, left heel raised

LUNGE/SQUAT COMBINATION

All exercises with a light body bar on your shoulders

1 10 x right-leg-back static lunges

2 5 x narrow squats (4 counts down, 4 counts up)

3 10 x left-leg-back static lunges

4 5 x narrow squats

5 10 x step-forward lunges (alternate right and left). Try to get your back knee almost to the floor and remember to keep your knees in line with your toes.

SQUAT LEG RAISES

All exercises with a body bar on its end on the floor in front of you. Press down on the bar to get you lower in the squat.

1 10 x squat leg raises to the right
10 x repeat to the left

2 5 x squat leg raises to the right
5 x repeat to the left

FRONT LEG RAISES

On your back, knees bent, feet flat on the floor

1 10 x front leg raises, right leg, toes pointed
Hold straight leg at the top. Flex and point the foot twice, then lower. Keep your left leg bent.
10 x repeat on left leg

2 Repeat with a flexed foot, flexing the foot as you raise the leg straight up and down.

3 10 x front leg raises, right leg, flexed foot
10 x repeat on left leg

WIDE-LEG-SQUAT/CALF-RAISE COMBINATION

All exercises with a light body bar on your shoulders

1 10 x wide leg squats

2 10 x quick calf raises with upright row

3 10 x wide leg squats (2 counts down, 2 counts up)

4 5 x calf raises (2 counts up, 2 counts down, with upright row)

5 5 x wide leg squats (4 counts down, hold for 4 counts, then 4 counts up)

LYING BRIDGE

1 Hold for 30 seconds.
10 x scoop your buttocks under, then push up until you are in a straight line from neck to knee again.

2 Hold for 30 seconds.
Lift your right leg straight off the floor, hold for 10 seconds. Make sure your buttocks don't drop and your body stays in a straight line.

3 Hold for 10 seconds.
10 x repeat scoop and push-up

4 Lift your left leg straight off the floor, hold for 10 seconds.
Bridge position, hold for 20 seconds.

THE PLANK

Hold for 10 seconds, rest then repeat twice.

T-STAND

Hold for 30 seconds, rest then repeat.
Repeat on the other side.

V-SIT

Lift one foot 3–6 in. (7.5–15 cm) off the floor.
Hold for 30 seconds.
Rest then repeat on the other side.

Stretch out your muscles, paying particular attention to your legs and buttocks.

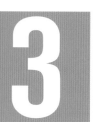

picking up the pace (cont.)

B BLOCK (30-MINUTE WORKOUT)

Start by lying on the floor, knees bent, feet flat on the floor

LEG RAISES

1 10 x leg raises. Keep your knees bent (alternate right and left legs).

2 10 x leg raises, both legs (4 counts up, 4 counts down)

RAINBOWS

Point your toes and lift your feet 2 in. (5 cm) off the floor.
10 x alternate to the left and right

SIT-UP/TRICEP-DIP COMBINATION

1 10 x sit-ups, hands by your ears
10 x tricep dips, buttocks off the floor

2 10 x sit-ups (2 counts up, 2 counts down)
10 x tricep dips, buttocks off the floor
(2 counts down, 2 counts up)

OBLIQUE-CURL/SIT-UP COMBINATION

1 10 x oblique curls (alternate right and left)

2 5 x sit-ups (4 counts up, hold for 4 counts, 4 counts down)
10 x quick oblique curls

3 10 x sit-ups (2 counts up, hold for 2 counts, 2 counts down)
10 x oblique curls with your hands in a low V (alternate right and left)

REVERSE-CURL/SIT-UP COMBINATION

1 10 x reverse curls
5 x sit-ups (4 counts up, 4 counts down)

2 10 x repeat reverse curls
10 x sit-ups

BACK-EXTENSION/PUSH-UP COMBINATION

1 10 x back extensions, hands by your ears

2 10 x push-ups
10 x repeat back extensions

3 10 x push-ups (2 counts down, 2 counts up)
10 x repeat back extensions

4 10 x tricep push-ups, hands underneath your shoulders
10 x repeat back extensions

DEAD-LIFT/SHOULDER COMBINATION

All exercises with a light body bar and the resistance band

1
10 x dead lift with the body bar (2 counts down, 2 counts up)
10 x behind neck press with the resistance band

2
5 x dead lift with the body bar (4 counts down, 4 counts up)
10 x shoulder press with the body bar (2 counts up, 2 counts down)

3
10 x dead lift with the body bar (2 counts down, 2 counts up)
10 x behind neck press with the resistance band

4
5 x dead lift with the body bar (4 counts down, 4 counts up)
10 x shoulder press with the body bar

BICEP-CURL/UPRIGHT-ROW COMBINATION

All exercises with the resistance band

1
5 x bicep curls, right arm
5 x repeat on left arm

2
10 x bicep curls, both arms

3
5 x upright row, right arm
5 x repeat on left arm

4
10 x upright row, both arms

5
10 x bicep curls, both arms (2 counts up, 2 counts down)

6
10 x upright row, both arms (2 counts up, 2 counts down)

how's it going?

During the leg raises, if your lower back starts to hurt, pull your abdominal muscles in more or go back to exercising one leg at a time until you feel stronger.

When practicing the bicep curl combination, if it is too difficult working both arms together, do one at a time. Also, do one arm at a time if you feel the lateral raise combination is too difficult.

LATERAL-RAISE/FRONT-RAISE COMBINATION

All exercises with the resistance band

1
5 x lateral raise, right arm. Stand to the left side of the band to make it easier.
5 x repeat on left arm

2
10 x lateral raise, both arms. If this is too difficult, repeat right and left arms separately.

3
5 x front raise, right arm
5 x repeat on left arm

4
10 x front raise, both arms

Stretch out your muscles, paying particular attention to your abdominals, arms, and back.

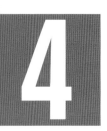

beginning sculpting

equipment

This level uses a wide range of equipment that will help to not only increase your knowledge but also vary your workout. However, you do not have to adhere rigidly to the recommendations here—feel free to choose your own equipment.

A BLOCK (30-MINUTE WORKOUT)

SQUATS

	All exercises with a medium body bar on your shoulders
1	10 x narrow squats 10 x narrow squats, right heel raised
2	10 x narrow squats, both feet flat on the floor 10 x narrow squats, left heel raised
3	Repeat the sequence (2 counts down, 2 counts up)

LUNGE/SQUAT COMBINATION

	All exercises with a medium body bar on your shoulders
1	10 x right-leg-back static lunges
2	5 x narrow squats (4 counts down, 4 counts up) 10 x left-leg-back static lunges
3	5 x narrow squats (4 counts down, hold for 4 counts, then 4 counts up) 10 x right-leg-back static lunges (2 counts down, 2 counts up)
4	5 x narrow squats (2 counts down, 2 counts up) 10 x left-leg-back static lunges (2 counts down, 2 counts up)
5	5 x narrow squats 10 x step-forward lunges (alternate right and left legs)

WIDE-LEG-SQUAT/CALF-RAISE COMBINATION

	All exercises with a medium body bar on your shoulders
1	10 x wide leg squats 10 x quick calf raises with bicep curl If you feel uncoordinated working your arms and legs at the same time, do the exercises separately. Put them together when you are more confident.
2	5 x calf raises with bicep curl (2 counts up, 2 counts down)
3	10 x wide leg squats (2 counts down, 2 counts up) 5 x repeat calf raises
4	10 x wide leg squats
5	5 x wide leg squats (4 counts down, 4 counts up)
6	Stay down in a wide squat. 10 x calf raises, right heel only 10 x repeat on left heel
7	10 x wide leg squats 10 x calf raises, both heels
8	5 x wide leg squats (4 counts down, 4 counts up)

SQUAT LEG RAISES

All exercises with a medium body bar on your shoulders

1 8 x squat leg raises to the right
8 x repeat to the left

2 4 x squat leg raises to the right
4 x repeat to the left

3 2 x squat leg raises to the right
2 x repeat to the left

4 8 x squat leg raises (alternate right and left)
Repeat sequence in reverse order.

LYING BRIDGE

1 Hold for 30 seconds.
10 x scoop your buttocks under, then push up until you are in a straight line from neck to knee again.

2 Hold for 30 seconds.
Lift your right leg straight off the floor, hold for 10 seconds.

3 5 x scoop your buttocks under, then push up until you are in a straight line from neck to knee. Lift your left leg straight off the floor, hold for 10 seconds.

4 Bridge position, hold for 10 seconds.
10 x repeat scoop and push up

5 Lift your right leg straight off the floor, hold for 10 seconds.

6 5 x repeat scoop and push up
Lift your right leg straight off the floor, hold for 10 seconds.

7 Bridge position, hold for 20 seconds.

LEG EXERCISE COMBINATION

All exercises with a medium body bar on your shoulders

Repeat the leg exercise combinations from level 3, see p. 77.

PLANK

Hold for 20 seconds, rest then repeat for 15 seconds; rest then repeat for 10 seconds.

T-STAND

1 Hold for 30 seconds.

2 5 x lower your hips down to the floor and push up (2 counts down, 2 counts up). Hold at the top for 10 seconds.

3 5 x lower your hips down to the floor and push up. Hold at the top for 10 seconds.

4 Rest then repeat on the other side.

V-SIT

Lift both feet 3–6 in. (7.5–15 cm) off the floor. Hold for 30 seconds.
2 x rest then repeat

Stretch out your muscles, paying particular attention to your legs and buttocks.

how's it going?

If you train at home and don't have all the equipment or if you find one piece of equipment more effective than another, feel free to improvise, or to simply go back to the more minimal amounts of equipment used in earlier levels. It is important that you feel comfortable with what you are using.

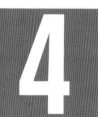

beginning sculpting (cont.)

B BLOCK (30-MINUTE WORKOUT)
Start by lying on the floor, knees bent, feet flat on the floor

LEG RAISES

1 10 x leg raises, both legs (4 counts up, 4 counts down)

2 30 seconds pedaling movement, alternating right and left leg. Keep your legs as low to the floor as possible.
If this hurts your lower back, pull your abs in more or go back to leg raises.

3 10 x repeat leg raises, both legs

RAINBOWS/REVERSE-CURL COMBINATION

1 5 x rainbows (4 counts down, 4 counts up)
10 x reverse curls

2 5 x rainbows
10 x reverse curls

3 5 x rainbows
5 x reverse curls

SIT-UPS

All exercises on the core stability ball

1 10 x sit-ups, hands by your ears

2 Come up into the sit-up position on the ball, with your arms in a low V-shape.
10 x oblique reaches

3 10 x sit-ups (2 counts up, 2 counts down)
Come up into the sit-up position on the ball, with your arms in a low V-shape.
10 x oblique reaches

4 5 x sit-ups (4 counts up, 4 counts down)
5–10 x sit-ups

TRICEP-DIP/OBLIQUE-CURL COMBINATION

Tricep dips with a light body bar placed across your hips; oblique curls on the floor

1 10 x tricep dips, with your buttocks off the floor
10 x left oblique curl, knees to the right

2 10 x tricep dips, with your buttocks off the floor (2 counts down, 2 counts up)
10 x right oblique curls, knees to the left

how's it going?

You may now start to notice changes in the tone of your muscles and in the amount of body fat you are carrying. However, different people progress at different rates, so do not be disillusioned if you find that improvements are not as noticeable as you had hoped. If you are progressing well, remember to keep working so you enjoy the results.

BACK-EXTENSION/PUSH-UP COMBINATION

1 10 x back extensions, hands by your ears

2 10 x full push-ups
10 x prone fly

3 10 x full push-ups (2 counts down,
2 counts up)
10 x prone fly

4 10 x full tricep push-ups, hands underneath
your shoulders

DEAD-LIFT/SHOULDER COMBINATION

All exercises with a medium body bar

1 10 x dead lift (2 counts down, 2 counts up)

2 10 x behind neck press
5 x repeat dead lift

3 10 x shoulder press and wide leg squats. Squat
down as you straighten your arms above you.

4 2 x wide leg squats traveling to the right
2 x repeat to the left

5 5 x dead lift (4 counts down, 4 counts up)
10 x behind neck press

6 5 x dead lift (4 counts down, 4 counts up)
10 x shoulder press and wide leg squats

BICEP-CURL/UPRIGHT-ROW COMBINATION

All exercises with a medium body bar

1 10 x bicep curls, both arms

2 5 x bicep curls, right arm only lifting the body
bar, left hand to balance it
5 x bicep curls, right arm only as before
(2 counts up, 2 counts down)

3 10 x bicep curls, both arms (2 counts up,
2 counts down)

4 5 x bicep curls, left arm only lifting the body
bar, right hand to balance it
5 x bicep curls, left arm only as before
(2 counts up, 2 counts down)

5 5 x upright rows, right arm only lifting the
body bar, left hand to balance it
5 x repeat on left arm

6 10 x upright rows, both arms

7 10 x bicep curls, both arms (2 counts up,
2 counts down)

8 10 x upright row, both arms (2 counts up,
2 counts down)

LATERAL-RAISE/FRONT-RAISE COMBINATION

All exercises with light hand weights

1 5 x lateral raise, right arm
5 x repeat on left arm

2 10 x lateral raise, both arms

3 5 x front raise, right arm
5 x repeat on left arm

4 10 x front raise, both arms

5 Repeat whole sequence.

Stretch out your muscles, paying particular attention to your abdominals, arms, and back.

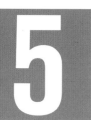

advanced sculpting and toning

growing confidence

By now you should be feeling more confident about the exercises in this program. You should also be getting stronger and ready to add heavier weights; however, do not worry if you are not. Instead you should stay at level 4 until you are ready to move up to this more demanding level. Remember, everyone builds muscle at a different rate.

changing shape

You may also have noticed differences in your muscle tone or body shape. If not, start to look at your nutrition and cardiovascular training. If you are building muscle but it is covered in a layer of fat then it will be hard to see the difference. To lose body fat, change your fitness program from the previous level to meet your new goals. Below left is a suggested training week.

MONDAY	A block (hips, legs, buttocks, and core muscles)
TUESDAY	30 minutes cardiovascular training (for example, jogging)
WEDNESDAY	B block (abs, arms, shoulders, chest, and back)
THURSDAY	30 minutes fat-burning exercise (for example, cycling)
FRIDAY	45-minute aerobic class
SATURDAY	30–45 minutes swimming
SUNDAY	Rest day

A BLOCK (30–45-MINUTE WORKOUT)

SQUATS

All exercises with a medium to heavy barbell on your shoulders

1	10 x narrow squats 10 x narrow squats, right heel raised
2	10 x narrow squats, both feet flat on the floor 10 x narrow squats, left heel raised
3	Repeat sequence (2 counts down, 2 counts up).

STATIC-LUNGE/SQUAT COMBINATION

All exercises with a medium to heavy barbell on your shoulders

1	10 x right-leg-back static lunges
2	5 x narrow squats (4 counts down, 4 counts up) 10 x left-leg-back static lunges
3	5 x narrow squats (4 counts down, hold for 4 counts, then 4 counts up) 10 x right-leg-back static lunges (2 counts down, 2 counts up)
4	5 x narrow squats (4 counts down, 4 counts up) 10 x left-leg-back static lunges (2 counts down, 2 counts up)
5	5 x narrow squats (2 counts down, 2 counts up)
6	10 x step-forward lunges, with upright row (alternate right and left legs)

WIDE-LEG-SQUAT/CALF-RAISE COMBINATION

All exercises with a medium to heavy barbell

1 10 x wide leg squats

2 10 x quick calf raises with bicep curl or upright row
5 x calf raises (2 counts up, 2 counts down) with bicep curl or upright row

3 10 x wide leg squats (2 counts down, 2 counts up)
5 x repeat calf raises

4 Go down into a wide leg squat with the barbell on your shoulders.
10 x calf raises lifting right heel, then left heel

5 10 x wide leg squats
5 x wide leg squats (4 counts down, 4 counts up)

SQUAT LEG RAISES

All exercises with a medium to heavy barbell

1 8 x squat leg raises to the right
8 x repeat to the left

2 4 x squat leg raises to the right
4 x repeat to the left

3 2 x squat leg raises to the right
2 x repeat to the left

4 8 x squat leg raises (alternate right and left legs)

5 Repeat sequence in reverse order.

LYING BRIDGE

All exercises on the core stability ball. Place the soles of your feet on the ball and your arms to the sides.

1 Hold for 30 seconds.
10 x scoop your buttocks under, then push up until you are in a straight line from neck to knee again.

2 Hold for 30 seconds.
Lift your right leg straight off the ball. Hold for 10 seconds.
Lower your leg, then hold the bridge for 10 seconds.

3 10 x repeat scoop and push up
Lift your left leg straight off the ball and hold for 10 seconds.
Lower your leg, then hold the bridge for 20 seconds.

PLANK

Hold for 30 seconds. Relax then repeat.

T-STAND

1 Hold for 30 seconds.
5 x lower your hips down to the floor and push up (2 counts down, 2 counts up). Hold at the top for 20 seconds.

2 5 x lower your hips down to the floor and push up. Hold at the top for 20 seconds.
Rest then repeat on the other side.

V-SIT

Hold for 30 seconds. Try to straighten one leg, then the other.
Rest then repeat twice.

Stretch out your muscles, paying particular attention to your legs and buttocks.

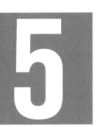

advanced sculpting and toning (cont.)

B BLOCK (30–45-MINUTE WORKOUT)
Start by lying on the floor

LEG-RAISE/RAINBOW COMBINATION
All exercises with the core stability ball gripped between your legs

1
5 x leg raises (4 counts up, 4 counts down)
5 x rainbows (4 counts down, 4 counts up)

2
5 x leg raises
5 x rainbows

REVERSE-CURL/RAINBOW COMBINATION
All exercises with the core stability ball gripped between your legs

1
5 x reverse curls
5 x rainbows

2
Repeat the sequence.

Finally, if you want to concentrate on building lean muscle tissue, you could alternate the A and B blocks every day of the week, combining them with aerobic training. Remember to have a day off for your muscles to repair themselves.

Monday	A block (hips, legs, buttocks, and core muscles)
Tuesday	B block (abs, arms, shoulders, chest, and back)
Wednesday	A block
Thursday	B block
Friday	A block
Saturday	B block
Sunday	Rest day

SIT-UP/OBLIQUE-REACH COMBINATION
All exercises on the core stability ball

1
10 x sit-ups, hands by your ears
Come up into the sit-up position on the ball, with your arms in a low V-shape.
10 x oblique reaches

2
10 x sit-ups (2 counts up, 2 counts down)
10 x oblique reaches, hands in a low V-shape

3
5 x sit-ups (4 counts up, hold for 4 counts, then 4 counts down)
5–10 x sit-ups

TRICEP-DIP/OBLIQUE-CURL COMBINATION
All exercises on the core stability ball

1
10 x tricep dips. Keep your buttocks as near to the ball as you can.
10 x oblique curls (count up, across, up, and down)

2
5 x tricep dips (2 counts down, 2 counts up)
10 x oblique curls

3
2 x tricep dips (4 counts down, 4 counts up)
10 x oblique curls

BACK-EXTENSION/PUSH-UP COMBINATION

All exercises on the core stability ball. Lay on your front on the ball, balancing on the balls of your feet.

1 10 x back extensions

2 Move forward on your hands, placing either your thighs (easiest), knees (intermediate), or ankles (advanced) on the ball.
10 x push-ups

3 Walk your hands back so that your feet are on the floor.
10 x prone fly or back extensions

4 Walk your hands forward to the first position.
5 x push-ups (2 counts down, 2 counts up)

5 Walk your hands back so that your feet are on the floor.
5 x prone fly or back extensions

6 Walk your hands forward to the first position.
5 x tricep push-ups, hands underneath your shoulders

DEAD-LIFT/SHOULDER COMBINATION

All exercises with a medium to heavy barbell or hand weights

1 10 x dead lift (2 counts down, 2 counts up)
5 x dead lift

2 10 x behind neck press
5 x repeat dead lift

3 10 x shoulder press
5 x dead lift (4 counts down, 4 counts up)

4 10 x behind neck press
5 x dead lift (4 counts up, 4 counts down)

5 10 x shoulder press

BICEP-CURL/UPRIGHT-ROW COMBINATION

All exercises with a medium to heavy barbell

1 10 x bicep curls
10 x upright row

2 5 x bicep curls (2 counts up, 2 counts down)
5 x upright row (2 counts up, 2 counts down)

3 5 x bicep curls (4 counts up, 4 counts down)
5 x upright row (4 counts up, 4 counts down)

4 5 x bicep curls
5 x upright row

LATERAL-RAISE/FRONT-RAISE COMBINATION

All exercises with light to medium hand weights

1 5 x lateral raise, right arm
5 x repeat on left arm

2 10 x lateral raise, both arms

3 5 x front raise, right arm
5 x repeat on left arm
10 x front raise, both arms

4 Repeat whole sequence.

Stretch out your muscles, paying particular attention to your abdominals, arms, and back.

how's it going?

If you are feeling physically tired, listen to your body and give yourself a day off—there is always tomorrow. However, if you are more mentally tired than physically tired, a workout can help get your mind off your stressors and leave you feeling better physically.

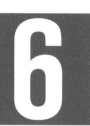

expert sculpting

You should now be able to create your own program to achieve your personal goals. It is best to cross-train, combining lots of different activities to get you fitter in every way. For example, you can run for CV fitness, do your A and B blocks for toning, do yoga to improve your suppleness, and play tennis to improve your coordination.

focus your training

You should be aware of what body part an exercise is working, how hard you are training, and how you can improve. Repeat sets for any body part you need to strengthen. You should feel confident using different equipment, and you should be able to adjust your program to work different muscles on different days.

WARM-UP

Now matter how experienced you are or how fit you are, you still need to warm up and stretch properly (see pp. 38–47).

A BLOCK (45-MINUTE WORKOUT)

SQUAT

All exercises with a medium or heavy barbell

1	10 x narrow squats
2	10 x narrow squats, right heel raised 10 x narrow squats, both feet flat on the floor 10 x narrow squats, left heel raised
3	Repeat whole sequence (2 counts down, 2 counts up)
4	Repeat whole sequence (4 counts down, 4 counts up)

STATIC–LUNGE/SQUAT COMBINATION

All exercises with a medium or heavy barbell

1	10 x right-leg-back static lunges 10 x narrow squats (2 counts down, 2 counts up) 10 x left-leg-back static lunges
2	5 x narrow squats (4 counts down, hold for 4 counts, then 4 counts up) 10 x right-leg-back static lunges (2 counts down, 2 counts up) 5 x narrow squats (4 counts down, hold for 4 counts, 4 counts up) 10 x left-leg-back static lunges (2 counts down, 2 counts up)
3	5 x narrow squats (2 counts down, 2 counts up) 3 x right-leg-back static lunges (4 counts down, 4 counts up) 5 x narrow squats 3 x left-leg-back static lunges (4 counts down, 4 counts up)
4	5 x narrow squats 10 x step-forward lunges with upright row (alternate right and left legs)

WIDE-LEG-SQUAT/CALF-RAISE COMBINATION

All exercises with a medium or heavy barbell

1 10 x wide leg squats
10 x quick calf raises with bicep curl or upright row

2 5 x calf raises (2 counts up, 2 counts down) with bicep curl or upright row
10 x wide leg squats (2 counts down, 2 counts up)
5 x repeat calf raises

3 Go down into a wide squat with the barbell on your shoulders.
10 x calf raise, right heel then left heel
10 x wide leg squats
5 x calf raises (2 counts up, 2 counts down) with bicep curl or upright row

4 Go down into a wide squat with the barbell on your shoulders.
6 x calf raise, right heel then left heel
5 x wide leg squats (4 counts down, 4 counts up)

SQUAT LEG RAISES

All exercises with a medium or heavy barbell

1 8 x squat leg raises to the right
8 x repeat to the left

2 4 x squat leg raises to the right
4 x repeat to the left

3 2 x squat leg raises to the right
2 x repeat to the left

4 8 x squat leg raises (alternate right and left legs)

5 Repeat whole sequence in reverse.

how's it going?

Be proud of what you have achieved so far and look forward to learning more so you can be fit for life. Ask yourself: Does it feel good to know that you are taking control of how you look? Do you feel stronger and fitter? This should now be having a positive impact on all aspects of your life.

LYING BRIDGE

All exercises on the core stability ball. Place your feet flat on the ball, legs straight, arms to the sides.

1 Hold for 30 seconds.

2 10 x scoop your buttocks under, then push up until you are in a straight line from neck to knee again.
Hold for 30 seconds.

3 Lift your right leg straight off the ball, hold for 15 seconds.
5 x scoop your buttocks under, then push up with your right leg still off the ball.
Hold for 15 seconds, with your right leg still off the ball.

4 Lower your right leg and hold the bridge position for 20 seconds.

5 Repeat step 3 on left leg.

6 Lower your left leg and hold the bridge position for 20 seconds.

PLANK

Hold for one minute. Lift one leg and hold for 10 seconds. Lower the leg, then lift the other leg. Rest then repeat, holding the plank position for 30 seconds.

T-STAND

1 Hold for 30 seconds and raise your top leg 6 in. (15 cm). Hold for 10 seconds then lower.

2 5 x lower your hips down to the floor and push up (2 counts down, 2 counts up). Hold at the top for 30 seconds.

3 10 x lower your hips down to the floor and push up. Hold at the top for 20 seconds. Rest then repeat on the other side.

V-SIT

Hold for 1 minute.
Straighten both legs and hold for 10 seconds. Rest then repeat twice, holding for 30 seconds.

Stretch out your muscles, paying particular attention to your legs and buttocks.

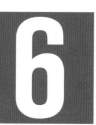

expert sculpting (cont.)

B BLOCK (45-MINUTE WORKOUT)
Start by lying on the floor

LEG-RAISE/RAINBOW COMBINATION

All exercises with the core stability ball gripped between your legs

1
10 x leg raises (4 counts down, 4 counts up)
10 x rainbows (4 counts down, 4 counts up)

2
10 x leg raises
10 x rainbows

REVERSE-CURL/RAINBOW COMBINATION

All exercises with the core stability ball gripped between your legs

1
10 x reverse curls
5 x rainbows

2
10 x repeat reverse curls
5 x rainbows

TRICEP-DIP/OBLIQUE-CURL COMBINATION

All exercises with the core stability ball and light body bar where specified

1
10 x tricep dips, the body bar across your hips. Keep your buttocks as near to the ball as you can.

2
10 x oblique curls
5 x tricep dips with the body bar (2 counts down, 2 counts up)

3
10 x oblique curls
2 x tricep dips with the body bar (4 counts down, 4 counts up)

4
10 x oblique curls

5
Repeat whole combination.

SIT-UP/OBLIQUE-REACH COMBINATION

All exercises on the core stability ball

1
10 x sit-ups, hands by your ears

2
Come up into the sit-up position on the ball with your arms in a low V-shape.
10 x oblique reaches

3
10 x sit-ups (2 counts up, 2 counts down)
10 x oblique reaches, hands in a low V-shape

4
5 x sit-ups (4 counts up, hold for 4 counts, then 4 counts down)

5
5–10 x sit-ups

6
Repeat whole combination.

BACK-EXTENSION/PUSH-UP COMBINATION

Lay on your front on the core stability ball, balancing on the balls of your feet

1 10 x back extensions. Move forward on your hands, placing either your knees (intermediate), or ankles (advanced) on the ball.

2 10 x push-ups with wide hands. Walk your hands back so that your feet are on the floor.

3 10 x prone fly or back extensions
Walk your hands forward to the first position.

4 10 x push-ups (2 counts down, 2 counts up)
Walk your hands back so that your feet are on the floor.

5 10 x prone fly or back extensions
Walk your hands forward to the first position.

6 10 x tricep push-ups, hands underneath your shoulders
Repeat whole combination.

DEAD-LIFT/SHOULDER COMBINATION

All exercises with a medium to heavy barbell or hand weights

1 10 x dead lift (2 counts down, 2 counts up)
5 x dead lift

2 10 x behind neck press
5 x repeat dead lift

3 10 x shoulder press
5 x dead lift (4 counts down, 4 counts up)

4 10 x behind neck press
5 x dead lift (4 counts up, 4 counts down)

5 10 x shoulder press

6 Repeat whole combination.

BICEP-CURL/UPRIGHT-ROW COMBINATION

All exercises with a medium to heavy barbell

1 10 x bicep curls
10 x upright row

2 10 x bicep curls (2 counts up, 2 counts down)
10 x upright row (2 counts up, 2 counts down)

3 5 x bicep curls (4 counts up, 4 counts down)
5 x upright row (4 counts up, 4 counts down)

4 10 x bicep curls
10 x upright row

5 Repeat whole combination.

LATERAL-RAISE COMBINATION

All exercises with medium hand weights

1 10 x lateral raise, right arm
10 x repeat on left arm

2 10 x lateral raise, both arms

3 10 x front raise, right arm
10 x repeat on left arm

4 Repeat whole combination.

Stretch out your muscles, paying particular attention to your abdominals, arms, and back.

continuing your program

You should now feel confident using a variety of equipment to give yourself a challenging total body workout. You have learned exercises that you can use in or out of the gym, on vacation, or even while watching television.

If you have been following a healthy eating program and have been incorporating aerobic training into your schedule, you should be seeing some improvement in your muscle strength, fat loss, and body tone. You should be feeling more coordinated and aware of which muscles the different exercises work. If you cannot feel an exercise working, go back to chapter three and check your technique in front of a mirror or a friend. If you still find some exercises harder than others, work at your own level until you feel ready to move on.

It is now your turn to create a program for yourself. Remember that,

MIX AND MATCH
Remember to warm up and stretch before your workout and to cool down and stretch afterward. Look back at all the exercises you have learned, and mix and match to ensure a varied and challenging workout.

TIPS ON BASIC TRAINING SO YOU CAN KEEP PROGRESSING

1 Do more repetitions of an exercise (15–25) at a lower weight for endurance training to improve your stamina.

2 Do fewer repetitions (1–12) of an exercise with a heavier weight for strength training.

3 Vary the rest time between sets or repetitions.

4 Change the rhythm or speed of an exercise. For example, you might execute a squat in one count rather than four counts.

5 Increase the weight or resistance of an exercise. You can do this by using different equipment.

6 Increase your range of movement by bending down farther to work harder on stretching exercises.

7 Change the intensity of your workout. For example, if you normally run for 10 minutes, you could jog more slowly for 25 minutes instead.

8 Change the frequency of your training by training three times a week instead of two.

9 Change the duration of your training session.

as your body gets used to training at a certain weight, for a certain time, or in a certain way, you will need to modify your training schedule to keep seeing results. As you get stronger and fitter you will have to add more weights or train for longer to make a difference.

muscles in mind

Try to train the largest muscle groups, like your legs, before smaller muscles, like your arms, which get tired more easily. Do not train the same muscle group on consecutive days, because your muscles need time to rest and repair themselves. When we overload our muscles we are actually damaging them, and it is during rest periods that they rebuild and grow stronger.

training schedule

Write down your schedule for the next week and leave it somewhere visible— for example, in your diary or on your fridge door. Make your schedule detailed so that you make time to train; it could look something like the training schedule below.

TRAINING SCHEDULE

MONDAY	Lunchtime aerobics class
TUESDAY	Abdominal and arm exercises at home after work
WEDNESDAY	Swimming (perhaps with the children after school)
THURSDAY	Hips, legs, and buttocks exercises at home after work
FRIDAY	Kickboxing or yoga class at lunch
SATURDAY	Roller skating or bike ride (the whole family can do this)
SUNDAY	Rest day

where do I go from here?

The best advice is to be brave and try new things. Look out for information on classes, groups, and gyms in your local area. You don't have to go back if an activity or class is not for you.

Make inquiries about what is on offer and go to watch classes before you start. However, be warned: lots of gyms now call their classes confusing things in an attempt to make them sound new or fashionable. Aerobics can be called anything from "funk-a-jam" to "aero blast," "spinning," "disco ride," or "road rally" and you may need to speak to the instructor in order to discover what each class actually involves.

To maintain your interest, exercise must be fun, rewarding, and sociable. So work out with partner and establish a reward system for reaching your goals. Or develop a positive relationship with experts at the gym who can suggest ways to help you have fun exercising. The following guide, which is by no means exhaustive, may give you a few ideas on activities that can reinvigorate your exercise routine.

OUTDOOR EXERCISE

When we spend so much time in offices, it is fantastic to be outside and to enjoy some space and scenery. It can also be a way of discovering new places and seeing new things.

ROLLER SKATING/BLADING
Look out for groups that meet in local parks. It's a great leg and buttocks workout.

CYCLING
It's environmentally friendly, great for your legs and heart, and for fat burning. You also notice things that you would drive straight past in a car.

POWER WALKING
Look out for clubs in your local area. It's a great way to get outdoors.

RUNNING OR JOGGING
It's one of the best cardiovascular, fat-burning, all-body workouts and it doesn't cost much money to get started.

CLIMBING
With proper supervision and safety equipment, climbing is one of the most rewarding forms of exercise. You will face a new challenge every time you climb, and you will also get a great upper-body workout.

WATER SPORTS
Have great fun getting out on the water by sailing, rowing, or canoeing. These are also great sports for meeting new people.

VOLLEYBALL, BASKETBALL, OR SOCCER
Local teams are usually grateful for new participants. Playing as a team is great fun and perfect for making new friends.

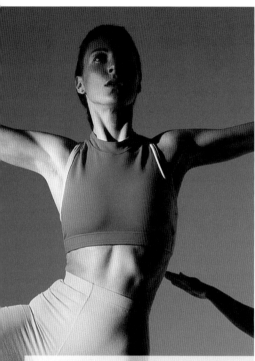

With so much to choose from how could you possibly get bored with getting fit? I hope the above has given you an insight into the wide variety of activities on offer. All you need to do is keep an open mind and be bold enough to try a few. If you can do this, you will continue to be fit, toned, healthy, and happy throughout all your life.

SWIMMING

A good all-over workout, but you will have to swim fast or for a long time to burn lots of calories.

STUDIO GYM CLASSES

AEROBICS
Perfect fat burning for those who get bored on running machines or stair climbers. You will get a 1-hour or 45-minute workout.

STEP CLASSES
Great for strengthening knees if done properly. Also good for burning fat and improving coordination.

BODY PUMP OR SCULPT CLASSES
Perfect for muscle building and toning, especially if you don't like training in a gym or find it hard to motivate yourself.

KICKBOXING/BOXING
Fantastic for upper-body definition and stress release. Also a good cardiovascular workout.

SPINNING
Probably the best fat-burning, cardiovascular workout. Will get your heart stronger very quickly. Also has anaerobic benefits.

AQUA
A low-impact form of exercise, perfect if you are new to fitness, recovering from an injury, or pregnant. Good fun and great for meeting new people.

HOLISTIC, MIND-BODY EXERCISES

YOGA
Very calming and relaxing but also challenging and great for stretching your muscles. Try different yoga classes depending on whether you want a workout or a more spiritual approach.

PILATES
Great for muscle toning and improving posture.

DANCE

SALSA CLASSES
Great for improving coordination and fat burning.

HIP-HOP/FUNK/STREET JAZZ DANCE CLASSES
Great for learning all those moves you see in pop videos.

index